"Just am...

"Thank you, Alison, for rising up off the bathroom floor and figuring out how to get out of that dark place us mamas so often find ourselves in. Thank you for showing us the light and that it does not have to be that way if our needs are met first! Who knew taking care of others starts with taking care of us?"

"An inspiration for all moms everywhere!"
- Marlene, mom and Kindergarten teacher

"Where was Alison when I was raising young children over a decade ago? Self-sacrificing to meet the needs of my family left me empty, drained, and beyond exhausted! Life for me included tears, doubt, and guilt. Alison has taught me how to set boundaries, how to love my family by first loving and caring for me, and how leading a healthy lifestyle leads to freedom and renewed energy. Alison's book is an inspiration for all moms everywhere!"

"What an inspirational piece of writing."
- Stacey, working mom of 2

"Her motivation has never been money or fame, Ali truly wants moms to live healthy and full lives. I mean it when I say you won't find anyone who is as real and raw as Alison. The true stories she will share in the coming pages will not only inspire but will also make you feel better about everything you are going through as a mom."

Making The Switch

How to put yourself first in a world that tells you not to.
A survival guide for busy moms.

ALISON BROWN

ISBN Paperback: 978-1-072364-98-6
Ebook: 978-1-64184-950-0

Dedication

To God, who has carried me when I couldn't carry myself.

To my husband and best friend, Graham, who has always come to the rescue when I needed him most and who shows me every day what true love is.

To my three boys—Andrew, Levi, and Zachary—for making me "mom" and giving me so many reasons to live, to laugh, and to love.

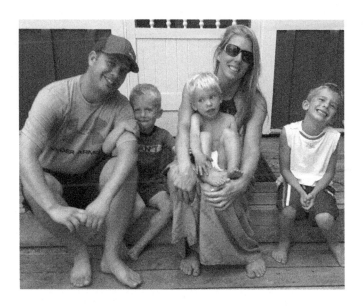

Table of Contents

Foreword

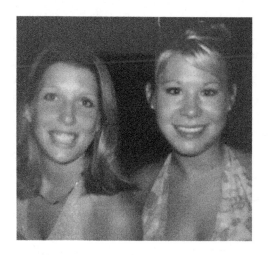

Picture this:
Two blonde twenty-somethings smuggling a blender into their university dorm to make healthy smoothies, while most of their roommates enjoyed fried foods at the campus all-you-can-eat buffet.

I first met Alison—Ali, as I most often call her—in Halifax where we both were about to begin an intensive journalism graduate degree program.

I was from the prairies and naively had my heart set on changing the world through television reporting. Ali's reason was far more personal and sincere. She was from a small town in Ontario called Walkerton. If the name sounds familiar, that's because it made headlines in 2000 across the globe when six people died from contaminated water. Alison saw firsthand the impact reporters could have on telling a tragic tale. She had a passion for writing, and after watching two thousand people, many friends and family, get sick from a water crisis, she decided to follow a career as a writer.

We bonded quickly with early morning workouts at the campus gym, making nutrient dense suppers on a camping stove in our dorm rooms, and running to a local boxing gym to get some cardio between classes.

Ali was always supportive and smart when it came to fitness. I have never told her this, but I often thought to myself, *What are you doing here? Sure, you are a talented writer, but you belong in a gym not a newsroom.* Her passion was and always will be fitness, health, and helping others live their best life, and as you read, you'll quickly see that she's amazing at it.

Her motivation has never been money or fame; Ali truly wants moms to live healthy and full lives. I mean it when I say that you won't find anyone who is as real and raw as Alison. The true stories she shares in the coming pages will not only inspire but will also make you feel better about everything you are going through as a mom.

We live in a world where far too many women feel the pressure to starve themselves the second their baby has left the womb. Our Instagram feeds are filled with moms making the perfect organic meal, working full time, and still keeping their picture perfect homes looking like something out of a magazine. It's no wonder many of us, including myself, are left to feel inadequate. That's why this book—this mommy movement, if you will—is so important. *Making the Switch* is helping women create happy lives, most importantly for themselves, but also for their families, too.

After the birth of my second child, I was tired. Actually, I was downright burnt out. My kids were not the best sleepers, and we were in the middle of building our home. I lived on coffee and felt like a shadow of my former self.

All it took was one phone call, and Alison got on a plane, left her babies at home, and came to my rescue. She made energy balls with whatever she found in my pantry and cheered me on while I fought back tears during basement work outs. She was there for me. She inspired me. And if you give her a chance, she will do the same for you. Now, turn the page and prepare to be inspired.

Stacey Ashley is a former television crime reporter turned public relations specialist, but most importantly, mom to Layla and Hudson.

Introduction

Mom Tired. It's a real thing.

There's a very big lie pervading mom world, and I am shamelessly embracing being a tattletaler. It's a lie that a good mom is a selfless mom. It's a lie that to be the best mom to your children you need to become a self-sacrificing human who shelves her own needs, and in their place, meets everyone else's. Let me tell you why we all must stop believing, and worse, living this lie.

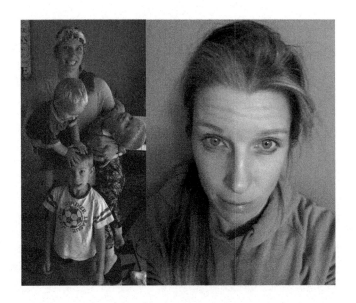

Moms everywhere are tired. I know this because I am a mom, and I used to be a very tired one. I also know this because I've worked with thousands of moms for many years, and when we first meet, tired roots run deep in every one of them.

I'm not talking about the kind of tired a kid-free weekend can fix, although that would certainly help. I'm talking about the kind of tired that leaves you so drained, so depleted, so exhausted that you feel as if you've got nothing left to give.

You get to the end of the day and feel like you couldn't possibly find a hint of energy for self-care, let alone exercise or food prep or house cleaning or even (especially!) a husband. And yet, somehow, moms still manage to find a way to tend to all of this and so much more, even though they are that tired.

Moms are empty, yet they keep pouring because they've been lead to believe that's what good moms do. They pour and pour until they look in the mirror and don't even recognize themselves. They yell at their kids and wish they wouldn't. Then they beat themselves up with guilt and regret for doing it. They have meltdowns they can't control. They are sad and resentful and angry and frustrated and lonely, but mostly, they're just tired; tired of living this lie and denying their own equally important needs.

Many moms feel desperate about their reflection in the mirror and the extra 10 to 30 or more pounds on the scale. Most moms are not who they used to be or who they want to be. They desire to have the energy and happiness they used to have so they can enjoy their kids rather than simply try to survive them. They give and give to everyone and everything else nonstop and leave nothing for themselves.

This "mom tired," as I like to call it, has an amazing solution that I have helped countless moms discover, including myself. It requires we all stop living the self-sacrificing lie. This lie is so prevalent that most moms believe it's in their very nature to be selfless, but I strongly disagree. I think the more we repress our own needs and desires for the sake of everyone else's, the worse we get for them and for us.

Guilt is supposed to be an emotional response to doing something wrong. This lie runs so deep that we are all believing it is actually a bad thing to put ourselves first. So bad that we have guilt for doing it. Think about that for a minute. Why should any mom feel guilty for tending to her needs? Since when did making yourself a priority become a bad thing to do? It's not.

There's a drastic yet simple switch that needs to happen to be free. Free from guilt and free from "mom tired" forever. A switch from being selfless to being selfish. I don't mean selfish in the negative sense of the word; I'm talking about a selfish that is actually completely necessary for your survival.

This switch is a process and requires several smaller switches to live healthily and be happy *with* children. The reward is you get to have your life and body back and be the role model you've always wanted to be and, quite frankly, the one you *deserve* to be.

Trust me, I've been where every tired mom is. I've gone through bouts of loneliness and depression. I've had yelling fits and mommy meltdowns and days where I look and feel like a "mombie." I've been disappointed with my post-baby body and wondered if I would ever get my life and body back. I've had guilt for taking time for myself and emotional outbursts for setting myself aside.

During my third pregnancy, I gained fifty-five pounds, and though my nine-pound baby boy and two older sons brought me so much joy, I was left sporting extra-large thighs, giant rolls in my midsection, saggy uncomfortable breasts, the weight of the world on my shoulders, and a tired feeling that went deep into my soul. In the back of my mind, I feared that this may be the way I look—and worse, feel—for the rest of my life.

I now had three small children to care for and couldn't be the mom I wanted to be. I was stuck in an exhausted fog of constantly cleaning my toddler's food off the floor, changing the baby's diapers, picking up a million Lego pieces that my oldest had left everywhere, drinking too much coffee, resenting my husband, and jumping to everyone else's call—in three different directions! I was setting myself aside and looking after everyone else because I thought that's what moms do.

From the minute that baby is growing inside of us, we are sacrificing. For some reason, I believed that once the child was born, that needed to continue. I thought that my needs, hopes, and dreams were no longer important. I actually believed that loving my kids meant setting myself and my wants and needs aside. Wow, was I ever wrong.

Shortly after having my third son, I had an epic meltdown (that I will share with you soon) that completely opened my eyes. For the first time, I saw the lie I was living. It was then that I took the steps I lay out in this book that completely changed my life for the better.

Now, I have the amazing privilege of helping moms everywhere make the switch from exhausted, burnt out, and unhappy with their bodies to energetic, healthy, confident, fit role models. Seeing moms get their happy back is incredible. Seeing kids get their mom back is beyond rewarding. Helping moms realize they don't have to run around empty any longer is life changing. Keep reading, and trust me, you too will be free.

Do not spend one more day of your life unhappy or unhealthy. Do not spend one more second trying to *survive* life with kids. Make the switch and get your happiness, your body, and your life back. You deserve this, and so do your children.

I invite you to come over to the happier, healthier, much less stressed side of mom life and bring your needs, your hopes, and your dreams with you because, from this moment on, they matter, too.

1

The Meltdown That Started This Movement

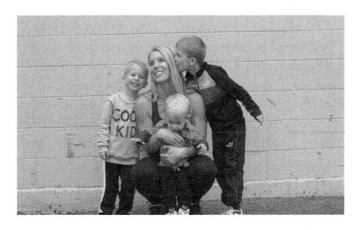

've had mommy meltdowns before, but this one was EPIC. It was a meltdown I know I will never forget, and likely my oldest child will, unfortunately, always remember as well. It's appropriate to say that it was the mother of all meltdowns, and though, at the time, I was worried it might damage my children permanently, in hindsight, it was the very thing that gave them their mother back.

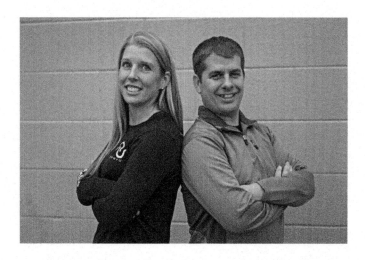

I have 3 sons: Zachary 2, Levi 5, and Andrew 7. They are all high-energy, active, full-of-life boys. My husband, Graham, and I have been in the fitness and nutrition industry for just over 20 years now, and we joke that to keep up with our 3 boys, we needed a 20-year head start in fitness to prepare us. Truthfully though, nothing could actually prepare us for what was coming.

Of those more than 20 years of operating fitness businesses, personal training, nutrition and weight loss coaching, and so much more, I've also been an athlete for 15 years. I thrive on the challenge of train-ing for a race or lifting competition. It's what keeps my energy up and my mental health in check. It helps me deal with stress, gives me some healthy "me" time, and keeps me strong enough to handle my 3 wild boys and whatever life throws our way.

I love fitness and healthy living with all my heart. It's amazing to get the opportunity to help others experience what it means to live healthier. It's so rewarding to be able to show people how they can look and feel their very best without having to spend hours exercising and without having to diet or deprive themselves of delicious food. Above all, I love showing them how great they can actually feel when they choose to make a lifestyle change and how that change can impact their entire family for the better.

Given my passion for fitness, you can imagine the devastation of being told I had to stop exercising several months after having my third son. I had just been given the green light a few months before, had a lot of weight to lose, and now was given the red. Exercise was how I was going to get my body back in shape, and it was also how I would mentally cope with the stress of running a business, a home, and raising three small children. I was devastated, to say the least.

Because my sweet baby Zachary was so big, my body couldn't accommodate his size, and it caused my abdominal wall to literally tear open while I was pregnant. The tear was so large that my belly button had become the size of a dinner plate. *I'm not even joking.* It shrunk down a little after he was born but was still large enough that a fist could easily fit into it. *Oh, the things our bodies endure.* Because of this, I was having severe lower back pain that had become debilitating. I sought out a pelvic health physiotherapist in hopes the back pain could be remedied, and I could get back to my training.

The physiotherapist told me I had come to her just in time. She was right. The abdominal separation had weakened my core so badly that it could have easily lead to a uterine prolapse that may have required surgery to fix. I needed to focus on closing the gap in my stomach and repairing my body from having such a large baby before jumping into a fitness program – *or before jumping at all or I'd be peeing my pants!* I was told I would need to stop exercising entirely and focus instead on the rehabilitation of my abdominal wall. Frustrating but necessary.

I didn't like what I heard but obviously listened because I understood the severity of the situation. I had worked with many clients who dealt with pelvic health challenges like these, and I knew mine needed immediate attention. These challenges are more common than you can imagine, and the good news is that if you are struggling with them, you don't have to. Most can be remedied if taken seriously and dealt with appropriately. *I promise you can get your body and your pelvic floor strength back mama.*

Listening meant that my post-baby weight loss was going to take a little longer and require I fine-tune my nutrition. Despite knowing what I needed to do nutritionally, I was left feeling disappointed that I couldn't exercise. I was very uncomfortable in my bigger-than-usual body and rather impatient and discouraged.

Because of my background, I was not only used to bouncing back to my previous fitness level and lean body fairly quickly after having babies, but I also had placed extra pressure on myself to do so. *Aren't we all very good at placing too much pressure on ourselves?* More on that later.

Truthfully, though, I was more than impatient and discouraged. I was getting angry and down about myself and the situation. It was slowly turning into depression. Exercise has been proven to be one of the best remedies for depression, and now I didn't have that daily dose of goodness I was used to getting.

I have no doubt the cause of my being down was not solely related to my delayed weight loss and halted exercise regime. It had to do with postpartum hormones, adjusting to life with three children, and trying to do it all on very little sleep without asking for any help. Along with the belief that I needed to be everything for everyone and set all my needs and wants aside, that was enough to put me over the edge.

On the day of my epic meltdown, I had been going a few months on no sleep. Zachary had just recovered from pneumonia and was not sleeping well, which left me extra tired all of the time. Extra tired for me usually left me short tempered with Andrew and Levi and extra emotional. Lack of sleep in combination with the selfless lie I was living was a recipe for disaster.

I remember the exact time of this meltdown because I was counting the minutes until Graham returned home from work to help take some of the load I was carrying. It was 4:00 p.m., and despite only having one more hour until he was home, I dreaded 4:00 p.m. every single day. For some reason, this felt like the hour that all hell was breaking loose in my home. I started to call it "hell hour." This seemed to be the hour that my kids misbehaved the most and with very little patience left, I almost always lost my cool. Today, though, I would lose my mind as well.

All three of my children were hungry, which meant blood sugar was low, which always makes them extra challenging to handle. I was doing my best to clean and cook dinner and cater to every call. I got them drinks and a small snack to tide them over until dinner was ready and was trying to entertain them while I held Zachary, who, since his birth, never wanted down and only wanted mom.

I distinctly remember the thought crossing my mind that I just wanted to sleep for days but instead of taking a five-minute sit-down break like I probably should have, I filled up a fourth cup of cold coffee, guzzled it down like a thirsty child, and continued to cook with the baby on my hip and a very tired soul.

It wasn't really one distinct incident or moment that set me off, it was a series of moments that escalated into a giant explosion. As I recall, my oldest son, Andrew, was bothering my middle son, Levi. This is a common occurrence in our home; some would call it brotherly love. Whatever it is, it drives me crazy on a good day. Levi was, of course, dishing it out just as much. The baby was crying because he needed to be fed, and I was racing to do everything for everyone all at the same time as all moms do. I was also asking, and more so, beating myself with questions like *Why am I no good at this mom thing?*

Someone spilled a cup of water, someone threw food across the table, the baby cried harder, and I raced to get him fed, which forced me to sit down and nurse him while my food boiled over on the stove and the other two fought.

The tipping point was Andrew and Levi's childish squabble escalating into a physical fight; a big one. Hitting and kicking was something that I had never witnessed before, and today was not the day for me to calmly break it up. Today, I yelled. I yelled and yelled until it became an out-of-control scream. I don't recall the words that came out of my mouth, but I do recall the stunned look on Andrew and Levi's faces as they immediately stood soldier still.

They were silent with their eyes wide open. Fear was all over their face, and tears came down mine like a flood that I couldn't hold back. The damn had broken. I angrily set the baby in the middle of the living room, turned the stove off, and then forcefully picked Andrew up and quite literally threw him into his room. I slammed the door so hard I almost broke it. Then I grabbed Levi and threw him on a step for a timeout. I had never been so loud or so rough with my children, and I honestly felt very out of control of my emotions and actions. It was like every frustration I had been bottling up for months unleashed in our home at that moment.

I carried myself and Zachary to the bathroom and locked the door. With a crying and no doubt terrified baby in my arms, I sat on the cold floor and called my husband's cell. He was my 911 that day and has been for many years. I am so thankful I even had someone I could call because I honestly don't want to know what would have happened had he not been there.

As the phone rang, I prayed he would answer it and be able to leave work early. Running our own business has a lot of demands, and he can't always leave on a whim, although this was clearly much more than a whim. By now, I could hear my no doubt traumatized boys outside my bathroom door crying and calling for me, begging me to come out.

Andrew is an extremely empathetic, beautifully sensitive boy, and I could hear him telling me he loved me and that he was sorry. Levi has a peaceful, soft-spoken personality that I knew had just been rattled. I can imagine my uncontrollable desperate sobs sounded horrible to them. I tried hard to control myself, but it felt impossible to hold back the flood. I reassured them I would be out soon and that everything was okay, even though it wasn't. I'm certain they already knew the truth—mommy was not okay at all.

Hearing Graham's voice on the phone temporarily calmed me down. Graham always has a way of doing that; it's one of the many things I love about him. I begged him to come home and explained that I was not okay. He could no doubt hear it in my voice despite me trying to hide it. A small sense of relief came over me knowing he was able to leave work early and save his kids from their mom. I felt horrible that they even needed saving, but I was in no place to care for anyone else. At this point, I was the one needing to be cared for.

While he was on his way, I sat on the cold bathroom floor in a complete state of misery for what seemed like forever. I held Zachary in my arms and stared into my floor-length mirror in anger at my saggy, overweight, uncomfortable body, crying about my life.

I wondered how on earth I got here. I was tired, sad, lonely, frustrated, angry, and every other emotion bad you can name. I felt an overwhelming sense of guilt about how I had treated my children just now, and I was beating myself up for my childish behavior—as if I needed another thing to feel bad about!

I wanted out, but I didn't really know what that even meant. It was not that I was suicidal, although I do fully understand how some moms can get to that place, and I completely sympathize with them. Hormones, lack of sleep, loneliness, stress, and the feeling of being completely overwhelmed can easily add up and make this "mom thing" feel like it's just too much to bear.

For me, it was more that I wanted relief from the exhaustion and deep sadness that came with the daily grind of diapers and cleaning and feeding and not sleeping and coffee and more coffee and being alone and tired with fussy kids all of the time. I wondered, *Is this what life with kids would be like for me forever? Was there not more to my life?* I had a career I wanted to get back to, and I felt stuck in a world and body I didn't want to be in but could not escape from.

I knew I needed something, but I had no idea what that something even was. I found myself entertaining thoughts of regretting having children if this was what having children was like. *Everyone makes it look so glamorous and fun. Everyone else appears to handle it much better than me. So many moms have it all together, and I don't. Why do I suck at this? Am I just not cut out to be a mom?* I then felt even more guilt for having such horrible thoughts. The truth was, I had this mom thing all wrong; I just didn't know it yet.

As I sat there crying, I missed the freedom that came with my old kid-free life. I missed my fit, lean body and fitting into my pre-baby clothes. I was so far away from fitting into them that I had piled them into boxes and hid them in the back of my closet so I wouldn't have to be reminded of how far I still had to go. Seeing them frustrated me. I missed being able to exercise. I missed conversing with adults. I missed having time for myself. I missed sleep. I missed feeling happy. I missed feeling like myself. Where did she go? I felt so lost and out of touch with who I even was anymore.

Somehow, every emotion and situation in my life culminated, and on that day, at that moment, I was *done* with living my life this way. Done, and yet I rationally knew I could never be done, and so I felt trapped, suffocated, isolated, and depressed all at once. I was so overwhelmed by the weight of caring for three kids and not caring for myself.

Hearing my kids announce, "Dad's home," gave me instant peace. I could hear the immediate calm in Andrew and Levi's voice. It felt as if a weight had just been lifted off of all of our shoulders. It had.

When Graham knocked at the bathroom door, I thanked God I didn't have to do this alone. To all of the moms out there who are, you are *amazing*, and you inspire me every single day. You are the true superheroes in mom world, and I hope you know it.

I opened the door and quickly handed him the baby. I continued to cry uncontrollably despite feeling some relief by his presence. When we made eye contact, he asked me what I needed, and more tears came flooding down. Though I didn't know the answer, the question itself made me feel totally supported and loved, and I certainly needed both at that moment.

It turns out that very question would be pivotal in me coming out of the dark place I had fallen in to. He stayed to hug me and then took the kids and left me alone where I wanted to be. As I sat on the bathroom floor, kid-free, crying like a child, I was overwhelmed by that question. Overwhelmed and terrified because I could not find the answer.

How could I not even know what I needed? How could I be that out of touch with myself? I knew I needed sleep, a kid-free shower, an adult conversation, and a day without bickering children, but I didn't know what I actually needed to become happy again, to feel good again, to feel like my old self again. I was so disconnected with what I needed to get back to me. The "me" I thought I was felt so far away. I felt lost.

Climbing out of that dark place took time and work and a lot of Graham's help and support. It was far from an overnight switch. I do not even know where I would be without Graham in my corner. His support was life-changing. He is skilled in a lot of areas, and mindset coaching happens to be one of them. I can imagine he never anticipated needing to work with his own wife when he studied in university, but I am so thankful he had these skills. His help, along with a lot of prayers, love, support, healing, exercise, healthy eating, and having my needs met, helped me find my way back home.

I started to ask myself that question on a daily basis. What do I need? What do I need today to feel good? What do I need to feel rested, calm, and happy? Am I getting what *I* need, too? Are my needs being prioritized the way I prioritize my children's and everyone else's? In all honesty, the realization that the floors being swept and laundry getting done were higher on my own list than I was, was eye-opening. Are my needs not more important than clean floors and folded laundry?

The truth was that I had been running around like a crazy person looking after everyone else's needs without having first met my own. Doing so eventually lead to the epic meltdown crash. Sometimes it takes crashing to realize something isn't working. I had no idea things needed to be fixed until I was broken on my bathroom floor.

In hindsight, this moment would be used to help thousands of moms come out of their dark places and find themselves again, and I must tell you that I am thankful for it. It was worth the sadness and the pain I went through because now something great has come from something awful. At the time, though, it was horrible.

Since sharing my difficult time with others, I am overwhelmed and saddened by the massive number of moms who are struggling in silence just like I was. We've all bought into the lie that we need to do everything for everyone else and set ourselves aside. We've all believed that a good mom doesn't need any help, that a good mom has it all together. Wrong.

The realization I had in my dark moment and the days and weeks that followed was that it was time for me to stop living the self-sacrificial lie and make a switch to being a healthy mom who puts her needs first and then meets the needs of her children second. Once I did this, so much changed. We all won.

There was a calm deep inside my soul that swept through our entire home. I yelled a lot less, I cried a lot less, I was happy for the first time in far too long. I was more patient. I was more grateful. I got to throw out my bigger clothes once and for all because I lost all 55 pounds and was in the best shape of my life. I had more energy, and above all, I felt like me again, the me I had lost when I became mom. I got my happy back, and my kids got the best version of me.

It wasn't long after things in my home got better that Graham and I both had this overwhelming sense of urgency to share this amazing switch with moms everywhere. We knew we had something completely life-changing that could impact moms and their families. Children deserve to have the very best of their mom, and moms deserve to be their very best. There's no better way to live life with kids.

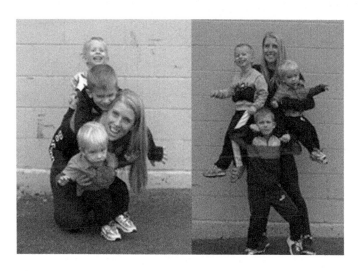

Moms can influence so many lives and impact the world in a major way, but first, they need to be liberated, loved, and have their needs met. Making the switch is the first step to incredible things happening in your home and your life, and if I can do it, so can you. Read on, and I will lay out exactly how you can prioritize yourself and come over to the better side of mom life, even if your hands are full and it feels like the weight of the world is on your shoulders.

2

Switch #1– The priority has to be YOU!

Why are moms tired? Why are postpartum depression and anxiety on the rise? Why is alcoholism so prevalent amongst thirty-somethings and growing at an alarming rate? To survive, moms are drinking coffee like it's water. Some are having Baileys for breakfast and mojitos for lunch. Most are reaching for wine to unwind at the end of the day.

Marketers have caught on. You can buy wine glasses that say "Mom's sippy cup" or bottles of wine that state "it's a pump and dump kind of day." Why are moms feeling too overwhelmed to cope with the challenges of raising children, running a home, going to work, being a wife, and whatever other demands they have on them?

I have no doubt there are thousands of studies supporting hundreds of different reasons why, and though I am certain they are all valid and offer some excellent insight, I know exactly why without having to research. I know why because I am a mom who had been there—tired, depressed, anxious, and an absolute emotional mess—until I, thankfully, made this switch.

I also know why because I've worked with countless moms, and every time we discuss making time for themselves, they are smacked in the face with the mom guilt door. They will sit at arenas, dance studios, and ball diamonds for hours, drive their children around the world, bust their butts preparing food, helping with homework, volunteering at schools and churches and community events, miss sleep, miss meals, throw amazing birthday parties and so much more, and they seriously battle with carving out even five minutes devoted to their needs. They would move the world for their children but struggle to lift a finger for themselves.

Every mom knows the age-old oxygen mask instructions given just before take-off; you must place your own oxygen mask on first before proceeding to help your children. The truth is, though, that every mom I have helped is not practicing these instructions. Heck, she, much like myself, doesn't even know where her own oxygen mask is, let alone how to put it on first!

She is running around like a crazy person just trying to survive. She prioritizes her children, her home, her husband, her friends, her family, her work, and everything else in her life above herself. Her needs are not even a thought in her mind. She doesn't know them because she is too busy meeting everyone else's.

Eventually this way of living forces the inevitable crash in the form of mommy meltdowns, irrational outbursts, exhaustion, anxiety, and depression. Many moms reach for alcohol, retail therapy, and coffee to cope. No one can live this way and thrive. No one can be healthy with this backward way of functioning.

We all know the oxygen mask needs to go on us first, or we will not be alive to help our children. For some reason, it's in our very nature to grab the mask and save our kids over ourselves. Why have we become so sacrificial? The cost is our own health, well-being, and happiness. The cost is that our kids get a burnt out, empty, irritable, and often irrational mom who's no good for anyone.

Now, please don't get me wrong here, given a real state of emergency, I would probably grab that mask and throw it on my children first, too, but in everyday life, here's what I know with absolute certainty: I cannot pour from an empty cup. Actually, let me rephrase that a little. I can pour from an empty cup, and so many moms are doing this, but no one gets anything good from a mom who's trying to pour from nothing.

In fact, when I am empty, I am the worst mom, wife, boss, friend, and family member. When I am empty, I am awful. I am cranky, I yell, I fight with my husband for no real valid reason, I feel resentful toward those I love, and my kids irritate the heck out of me. When I am empty, it's time to fill up, recharge, and make space for myself so that everyone that needs and loves me can get the best me and not the worst me.

The good news is that the more I work at it, the less often I even get empty. I've come to learn the signs that I am low, and I know just what I need to refill. Sometimes it's sleep, sometimes five minutes of putting my feet up, sometimes a good sweaty workout or a healthy sit-down meal, and sometimes all of the above in the same day. Whatever it is, I have come to learn to do it before I am empty. Most days.

Occasionally, though, life gets the best of me, and I lose my cool. Yes, I am still human. Unapologetically so. As you well know, children have a way of pushing every button you have all at the same time. Yesterday, as I was writing this, we were driving home from a beach day, and I was fully human. Levi and Andrew were on each other's last nerve and mine. Everyone was tired. As they bickered, I could feel my blood pressure rising. I was trying very hard to listen to a motivational speaker on my phone, and I couldn't hear a word. (In hindsight, I really should have had earphones) *Lesson learned.*

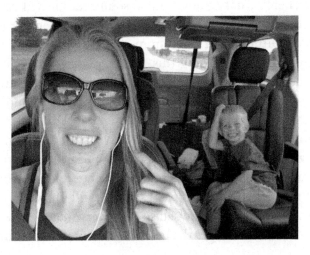

The tipping point for me was that my sweet Levi was so worked up that he went into a full-blown temper tantrum. The kid has a high pitched squeal that even the Chipmunks couldn't match. On most days, it's absolutely adorable. Today, not so much.

I was at my limit, and Graham was hoping and expecting I would calm myself down as a reasonable, grown adult should. He was about to intervene and stop the van to take some toys away from the boys when I lost it. I joined Levi and threw an adult temper tantrum, yelling and screaming and telling everyone to shut up. Not cool, but I own it. We all have days like this, no matter how much we work at being better. The good news is that I no longer feel guilty for overreacting, and I refuse to beat myself up for it. That's progress. Thankfully, these moments are much fewer and further between. That's progress, too. I'm working on it all, but of course, I am still learning.

If you can relate to being last on your own priority list and feeling exhausted and at the end of your own rope, you are not alone. If you are ready to enjoy life with kids rather than simply trying to survive it, please listen carefully. From this moment forward, you must be a little bit selfish, maybe even a lot. You must also live guilt free. I give you full permission to liberate yourself and your life and make yourself a priority on your own priority list. *The* priority. It's time to put your own oxygen mask on first, Mom, meet your own needs, cater and run around after yourself. It's time to take time out for you first. This is completely necessary for your survival, your happiness, and your longevity. It will make everything better, including your life with kids.

When my husband and I first started the Switch project—an online program exclusively for busy moms designed to help them make this switch from being last on their own priority list to being first where they belong—I had a mom named Annie who was amazed on the morning of day one.

She has two boys, and like most moms, her mornings were centered around them. She woke up and started her day by making their breakfast and getting them ready for school. On this particular day, day one of the program, she instead began her day with a short workout. She told her boys that she was first today, and they would get breakfast very soon, but they would simply have to wait and play quietly until she was ready to make it. Yay Mom!

While she worked hard and put herself and her health first, her boys went into the kitchen and got themselves breakfast. It turns out they were fully capable of getting their own breakfast; they just needed the opportunity to do it.

The lesson to all moms? Maybe you are holding your child back by putting them first all of the time. Maybe they are capable of more than you realize. Maybe they simply need to be given a chance to exercise a little independence. Maybe you need to take your hands off the wheel once in a while and let your children learn the skills that will help them succeed in life because, in life, no one is going to do everything for them. The best part? Making yourself a priority liberates not only you but also your children. Imagine the sense of accomplishment Annie's boys had when they were empowered to help themselves.

I was so proud of Annie and so thankful she was willing to share this story with all of our other moms and all of you. I have no doubt it took bravery and strength to step out of that old pattern and embrace this new life of putting herself first for a change. I know it's not easy, but I also know it's totally worth it.

To finish the story, these boys were, as I said, very proud of themselves and what they had accomplished. It allowed Annie to realize she perhaps had been doing more than she actually needed to be doing and could do a bit less. It also allowed her to get a great, twenty-minute, energetic start to her day, an all-around win.

I understand that life sometimes presents situations where you need to be selfless. If your child is sick, obviously you need to care for them and put their needs first. Even so, it's important you understand that, if your child is sick, you still need to eat and sleep and have five minutes of quiet time to recharge so you can care for them fully charged and healthy. Having sick kids can be draining, and if you do not care for yourself in the process, even debilitating. Trust me, I know.

When my oldest son Andrew was three, he almost died. The week before he was hospitalized, I noticed he was looking rather pale. That was it. There was nothing else out of character aside from being a little moody, which I attributed to lack of sleep and a typical three-year-old adjusting to his now-mobile younger brother.

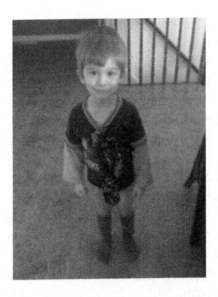

Andrew age 3 the day before we found out he was very sick.

Because of my past experience with anemia, I simply thought his iron levels were low. I happened to have a doctor's appointment booked to check my iron levels, so I decided to take him with me. This decision may very well have saved his life.

When our family doctor saw him, he reassured me that we likely had nothing to worry about. Andrew was running around full of life and energy, climbing on the hospital bed, and swiveling on the doctor's stool, just like his usual self. Our doctor ordered the blood work because he agreed that Andrew looked very pale.

At 10:00 that night, Graham got a call from a lab tech at the hospital telling us to get Andrew into the Emergency Room as fast as possible. She said he needed medical attention right away.

Graham, being the calm, uneasily shaken man that he is, asked the lab tech if she was certain we needed to wake Andrew up and take him to the hospital in the middle of a snowstorm. He was hoping it could wait until the morning, and so was I. We were both hoping it wasn't as serious as it sounded.

She insisted this was an emergency and that we needed to get Andrew help right away. His hemoglobin was at a 38, and he could die if we didn't move fast. The average healthy hemoglobin for a child at his age is well over 100. Andrew was not okay.

My heart sank as my mind went to all of the worst-case scenarios. A few years before Andrew was born, I had almost lost Graham to a freak accident. My heart was back to that moment, and my head told me this would be even worse. I was terrified.

We decided I would stay home with Levi who was sleeping while Graham raced half-asleep Andrew up the road to our local hospital. We both hoped this was a false alarm, but it wasn't. The doctor was in shock at the report of his hemoglobin levels and ran more bloodwork to be sure. The second report confirmed our fears; Andrew was in trouble. We were sent to the London, Ontario hospital for further investigation.

This was over an hour drive through a snowstorm, and Graham insisted he be the one to do the drive. Everything in me wanted to go with them and be there for Andrew, but by now it was midnight, the storm was even worse, and there was no way we could get childcare for Levi. I had to let them go.

As he packed things up to head to London, I will never forget Andrew's words. I leaned over to get him into the car seat and hugged him as tight as I could. I was trying hard to fight back tears because I didn't want him to worry. He then placed his hand on my arm and told me, "Don't worry, Mommy. God is with me, and I will be okay." Much like his dad, our Andrew has a way with words, and he brought me some calm in that very terrifying moment. Tears filled the corners of my eyes as I closed the van door, then my eyes blurred and the floodgates opened.

I wanted to believe that just as Graham had survived his near-death scare, Andrew would, too. As I watched the van pull away with what felt like my heart inside it, I was fighting hard to hang on to that hope. Standing in the freezing cold, watching snow circle around me I stopped trying to be strong and broke down into inconsolable sobs. I felt alone and so out of control. I begged God to save my child.

I was desperate and wanted more than anything to be with him. I would meet them in the morning, but until then, I wouldn't sleep a wink. A helpless, out-of-control feeling that was all too familiar flooded over me. Fear stole my thoughts and filled my body with adrenalin all night long. Despite having faith in God and a firm belief that everything happens for a reason, the thought of losing my child shook my entire world. *What if he dies and I never hug him again? What if he doesn't make it and that was my last goodbye? Maybe I should have gone with him. How could I have not gone with him?* These thoughts and countless others stole my sleep that night.

The days ahead were exhausting. Lots of testing finally landed us in oncology, and I feared the absolute worst—cancer. Thankfully, after many more tests and what felt like days of waiting, cancer was ruled out, but a bone marrow transplant was still on the table. We were sent to the hematology specialist where we learned that Andrew had a rare blood disorder called TEC (transient erythroblastopenea of childhood). Essentially, something stopped his bone marrow from working. To this day, they don't know what caused it, but because of this, he was slowly losing red blood cells. He was dying of oxygen deprivation.

Because of the lack of oxygen, his heart had developed a murmur to keep up. He had the lowest functional hemoglobin score any of the doctors had ever seen. He was still running around and seemed to have energy even though his skin was now a pale yellow. They couldn't believe he wasn't in the fetal position laying in a bed but speculated that Andrew's body had kept moving to keep his blood flowing faster, and therefore, his oxygen circulating to where it needed to be. They also told us his heart would have likely given out first. The body can only compensate for so long. We were very thankful Andrew's heart was as strong as it was because it was currently over-pumping to keep him alive.

I remember calling everyone I know and posting on social media asking for prayers for Andrew. The thought of not having him with us anymore was unbearable. As much as I wanted to be in control, I knew I wasn't. As I share this with you, I'm taken back to the intense shock, fear, and helplessness I felt as I witnessed my beautiful child endure needle after needle after needle. Sometimes, they would have to hold him down. Many times, despite our best efforts, he would cry.

The most heartbreaking was that I couldn't protect him from it, and I desperately wanted to be able to. At the time, he called them "pokeys" and would beg me with his big green eyes and very tired plea, "Please, no more pokeys, Mommy" to which I wanted to wrap my arms around him and promise him no more, but I couldn't make that promise and that broke my heart.

As moms, we have this intense desire to protect our children. It's in our nature to want to prevent our children from experiencing any pain, sadness, failure, or grief. It's funny that our nature is to protect them, yet to allow them to fail and experience pain and sadness and the many challenges of life is how they learn and grow and appreciate the good things life has to offer. Sometimes, we need to let go.

Our nature is to bubble-wrap our kids, yet bubble-wrapping them isn't healthy for them. It protects us from having to witness them in pain but prevents them from learning and growing the way they need to. At this moment, I couldn't do what I naturally wanted to do. All I could do was pray for Andrew and be there to hold him while he navigated this new experience and showed us how tremendously brave he truly was.

Andrew needed blood transfusions to get more oxygen and blood into his body. They had to break them up into smaller amounts of transfusions so his heart wouldn't get overloaded and fail. The hope was that more blood would get his bone marrow working again and put this whole thing behind us.

As we waited by his bedside watching a blood donor's blood save his life and praying that Andrew wouldn't have any allergic reactions to the new blood, Graham looked at me with deep concern. "You haven't slept for days, and I get that, but you also haven't eaten much. You need to eat, Alison."

Of course, he was right. It was then that I realized how hungry I actually was. It was also then that I had this amazing realization; I hadn't taken care of myself at all for four days straight: no sleep, very little food, barely any water, no shower, and constant worrying. It was awful. I was on a fast train to total derailment in the middle of our crisis. Had I kept going like this, I wouldn't be able to care for anyone. I would be the one needing to be cared for.

Realizing that if I was going to be healthy for Andrew, I needed to start taking care of myself, was so important. It wasn't easy to leave his bedside to eat and rest and shower. At times, I feared taking one second away from him. My mind would race to thoughts like, *What if he were to die, and I wasn't there beside him?* I had to force myself past these fears and take this very important time so I could come back rested, much more level-headed, and in a better state to be able to make good decisions. Graham and I worked as a team to ensure Andrew was getting everything he needed, and that we were too. Levi was in good hands with loved ones so we could focus our energy where it needed to be at that moment.

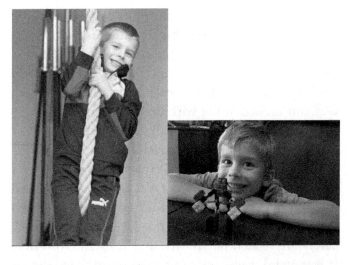

The great news is that the blood transfusions got Andrew's bone marrow working again, and as I write this, he is a happy, healthy, very energetic 7-year-old with a hemoglobin of 134. I am so thankful that he is still with us. I am thankful for blood donors. I am thankful for our family doctor and all of the great doctors and nurses and personal support workers who helped us navigate this scary time.

I am thankful for all that the Ronald McDonald House does to help children and their families at the London Ontario hospital. I am thankful for all of the prayers and support that kept coming from loved ones and even strangers during this intensely challenging time. Most of all, I am thankful to God for saving my son's life. I can't imagine life without my Andrew in it. He fills my heart with so much love and brings a world of excitement to each new day.

The night he received his last blood transfusion, there was no room for us to stay over. The hospital wanted to keep us close, so they put us up in a hotel. Andrew was feeling and looking much better. After ordering our dinner in, taking him to the hotel gift shop to get him a special toy (he picked out a bouncy ball), and then tucking him into bed, he looked over at Graham and I and spoke words I will never forget. "This is the *best* day ever!" My heart sank. For me, this was one of the worst days and few weeks of my life. At the time, I could think of so many better days, but in hindsight, he was right. We didn't actually know it then, but that was the day he was finally okay, and getting him back again made it the very best day.

Since this challenging time, and having come too close to losing Graham as well, I find myself often more aware of the fragility of life. Graham's freak accident involved him getting his hand caught in an indoor cycling bike chain. He was doing some maintenance at the gym we ran, and (brace yourself) when his hand made it through to the other side of the 45-pound flywheel of an indoor cycling bike, what he felt was a break was actually the loss of all 4 fingers on his right hand.

He needed emergency surgery to fix his hand (they were able to re-attach 2 fingers), and though he came through surgery strong, he was accidentally given too much morphine, which caused his lungs to stop working. He coded and came much too close to not making it. We had only been married a few years at this point and almost losing him was absolutely terrifying and completely life-altering. (I'm forever very thankful to a small group of wonderful people who were at the gym that day and helped Graham while I raced to meet him at the hospital.)

As much as I do not love to revisit the heart-wrenching emotions these moments bring back, especially the awful feeling of helplessness that comes with being out of control of the situation, I do love the reminder of what a blessing Graham and Andrew are in my life. On the hard days, that reminder allows me to be much more patient and appreciative of everyone in my life.

When our children are sick or going through challenging times, we so quickly set ourselves aside, but we cannot do this. We can't do this when they are sick, and we can't do this when they are healthy. We need to be a priority to be effective and good for everyone that needs and loves us.

This is not an easy switch. Every day will present its own set of challenges. I remember finally getting the green light to exercise again after working with the physiotherapist to correct my abdominal injury. Of course, I was elated, but when I first started trying to carve out time for myself to do it, I felt like everything was against me. It was as if my children were prompted to cry and beg me to stay and throw temper tantrums at the exact moment I was feeling guilty about leaving them. This made making myself a priority extra difficult.

I remember looking into Levi's tear-filled eyes and telling him (and myself) that I would only be gone for twenty minutes. Closing the door of my home and walking away was heart-wrenching, and at that moment, I felt as if I was fighting everything in me just to turn around and forget about my run for the day. But why should I set myself aside like that? I need that time to be good for Levi and everyone that loves me. He deserves that, and so do I.

Deciding to do it anyway was the hardest but best thing I could have ever done. I came back with a clear head, less stress, and a newfound calm. I was excited to see my boys again and felt energized for the entire rest of my day. The repetitive days didn't feel quite as difficult when I had taken time for myself. The more I did it anyway, the easier it became. The feeling afterward was always worth the struggle before.

Some days, making yourself a priority may simply be taking five minutes to put your feet up. Some days, it will be having lunch with a friend, taking a kid-free shower, or getting a workout in. Some days, it will be a spa day or getting your hair or nails done. Whatever it is, big or small, it's completely necessary.

You may have to get your husband to parent while you get this time for yourself. You may have to call a relative or a sitter or a friend. You'll need to learn to ask for help, and you'll also need to learn not to feel bad about needing that help. As moms, we seem to think we need to be able to do it all. This is another lie. We are human, and humans cannot do it all. In fact, we were never meant to. There's a reason the expression, "It takes a village" exists. That's because it's true. Being a mom and raising humans is the hardest job on this planet. We all need each other's help. Asking for it isn't a sign of weakness, it's a sign of strength and bravery.

As I am writing about getting help, one of our rock-star Switch moms posted to our group that she had just done a workout. She thanked her mom for the help and wrote, "I always felt guilty before when asking for help, but now I realize it never hurts to ask for a little help if you need it to complete something for you and make you better for everyone." What a tremendous realization! Instead of guilt, we should all feel a sense of pride in knowing we are strong enough to ask for help when we need it.

I can't promise you perfect, guilt-free days all of the time, but I can promise you that the more you do it, the easier and better it will get. You will be happier and healthier when you make this switch. The trickle-down effect is that your entire family will get the very best of you, and they deserve that just as much as you do.

Your children will be what they see. This really is true. They will not mimic what they hear, they will not become what you tell them, they will become what you show them. As they see a mom who is prioritizing herself, they will grow up knowing the importance of doing the same for themselves. What an amazing skill to have. Making this switch will give your child or children the skills they need to put themselves first. It will liberate you both. You owe it to them and yourself to make *you* a priority. Do it now. Do it for them, but above all, do it for you.

ACTION ITEMS:

Make yourself a priority! Start by carving out five minutes to enjoy your coffee or tea in peace.

Do something for yourself every day. Aim to do at least one thing for yourself every day (big or small, it counts). Note: This may mean laundry, countertops, and floors have to be set aside temporarily. Trust me, they will wait for you!

Pause and get in touch with your needs. When we jump to cater to everyone else's needs and plow into the busyness of the day without pausing, we often lose touch with our own needs. Before the day's race begins, ask yourself, "What are my needs, and how can I ensure they will be met?"

Sometimes, this is simply covering the basics like showering, drinking enough water, and eating enough healthy food. Sometimes, this means a workout, time away with friends, a massage, or a kid-free afternoon. Whatever your needs are, do your very best to first get in touch with them and then meet them as often as you can manage.

Ask for help. It's not a sign of weakness to need help, it's a sign of strength. It's so important that you don't try to do everything on your own. Get cleaning help, get childcare help, and remember, even twenty minutes can be enough. Every little bit counts.

Let go of all guilt from this moment on. Remember, it's not selfish to do something for you; it's completely necessary, and you will be better for everyone that loves you when you do it. The more you do this, the easier it will get, and pretty soon you'll replace feelings of guilt with feelings of gratitude for getting the chance to re-fill and come back ready to give from a very full cup.

3

Switch #2–You Must Love Yourself First!

I bet if I asked you to make a list of everything you dislike about your body, your personality, your life, and your ability as a mom, you could give me one heck of a list. Just a guess, but I suspect that asking for a list of everything you love about your body, yourself, and your ability as a mom would be shorter and much more challenging to compile. This has to change. Now.

Part of making yourself a priority is establishing the solid foundation that you matter. This requires breaking down the current foundation that exists inside of you. You will need to examine how you really feel about yourself and come to the realization of the truth that you have value—massive value! You are worth being a priority. You are special. You are beautiful. You are important. In fact, I would argue that you are the most important person, especially in your child's life. Therefore, it goes without saying that you need to love yourself just as much as they do, if not more.

To clarify, when I say you need to love yourself, I am not speaking in a negative context. I'm not telling you to walk around prideful and conceited. I'm saying you need to love yourself enough to care for yourself, to fuel your body healthily, to move your body often as it was designed to do, to rest it when it needs rest, to focus on gratitude and mindfulness and what kinds of things you are entertaining and allowing into your mind. You need to love yourself enough to be in tune with your needs and stop shelving them, like I was, until you don't even know what they are anymore, or worse, until you crash.

Can you look in the mirror and love your body? Can you stare at the body you are in and tell yourself you are beautiful? Can you list all of the amazing attributes, talents, and skills that you have and all of the value you bring to your community, workplace, home, family, and friends? Can you see that you are an important person to your children and loved ones? Can you believe in yourself and your value? You need to work on loving yourself this very moment with all of your beautiful flaws and amazing imperfections, and when you do, a whole lot will change for you for the better. This really is the most important skill you can learn.

It's time to get real with what you're telling yourself. What thoughts cross your mind regularly? What flaws do you point out about yourself? What negative self-talk do you entertain? How often in a day do you beat yourself up with guilt and regret? How often do you feel not good enough, inadequate, or insufficient?

Insufficiency is not a feeling that occurs because you actually are insufficient. It occurs because you've let your thoughts convince you that you are. The thoughts you allow to manifest will be what you become. The age-old expression that you are what you think you are really is the truth. So, what do you think you are? What are you saying to yourself that you are?

You would never tell your child what you say to yourself on a daily basis. If you were to stare into the face of your beautiful child, would you ever consider telling them they are fat or ugly or not good enough or a failure? Or how about that they suck at being a child? No way! In fact, you would hunt down and mama-bear-attack anyone who ever spoke an ill word toward your child, and rightfully so.

Why then, if you would never say these things to others, is it okay to say these things to yourself? Are you not just as important as a precious child? Are you not just as human, just as special, just as fragile, just as valuable? You are. Do you really stink at being a mom, or are you actually trying your very best? I bet you are trying your best. Why do you not attack the voice that says these horrible things to you? Why is it so hard to talk about what is great about you and easy to tell others what you wish you could change?

Most moms I start working with have a hard time with self-love. In fact, it makes them uncomfortable when I even mention giving me a list of what they love about themselves. They stumble and struggle to find positive words. In mere seconds, they can give me a massive list of negative things they would like changed about themselves, their bodies, and their abilities as a mom.

Here's the truth; it's perfectly okay to want to change your body, improve your health, and better yourself. It's excellent to want to get better at this mom thing. It's okay to want to lose weight. I help people do this every single day. It's a healthy thing to do. What is not okay is approaching weight loss or any goal about yourself from a place of hatred rather than love.

Getting stronger, leaner, healthier, more fit, coloring your hair and nails, going shopping for a nice new outfit, buying a self-help book, or investing in courses to improve yourself are all great things to do if they are done out of love. Doing them from a place of "I hate myself, so I need to change myself" is not okay.

Instead, it needs to be "Because I love myself, I am going to take care of myself, and that means caring for my body and my mind." I know this is easier said than done, but I promise it is not at all impossible. I am living proof, and so are all of the amazing moms I work with every day.

If you find self-love challenging, you are not alone. I used to struggle with all of this, too. Telling you that I didn't always love myself would be a massive understatement. In fact, self-hatred almost killed me, literally.

I grew up with an intense loathing for myself and my body. The negative comments about my looks started when I was very young. In most cases, I don't remember who from, but I do remember an immediate feeling of inadequacy and ugliness.

The first memory I have of disliking myself was with my cowlick that made my bangs stick straight up in the air. I vaguely remember a hairdresser simply stating the obvious, that I had a cowlick. That was all it took. I remember being very self-conscious from that moment on. I distinctly recall it starting at age six on picture day and for many years after that.

A few years later, my smile needed to be "fixed" because my lip came up high revealing my pearly whites and their gums a little too much more than "normal." A dentist actually said that my "gummy smile needed fixing." For some reason, this was just enough to give me a complex about my smile. I remember getting pictures taken from then on and not wanting to fully smile just in case it would look gummy and therefore, ugly in my mind.

I never got the surgery he suggested because there was a risk that if he hit a particular nerve in my face, I would never smile again. I decided that I would rather have a gummy smile then risk not having one at all.

The bridge of my nose has a bump that I remember disliking around this age as well. I had many people point it out to me. I recall wanting to get it removed and even looked into the cost and process. In the end, I never went ahead with that surgery either but with a cowlick, a bump on my nose, and a gummy smile, I went into my teenage years severely hating my face. Unfortunately, these insecurities stayed with me for many years after this, and pictures became something I hated getting taken and often avoided.

You can imagine my self-esteem when puberty hit, and I suddenly had a pair of large breasts, thighs, and hips to match. By then, I was fifteen pounds overweight and had a loathing for my body and my face. I recall adding a hatred for my legs to the growing list. I called them "tree trunks" and "heifer thighs" and covered them up as much as I could. I can't remember wearing shorts, a skirt, or a dress during most of my adolescent years, unless they were long. Basketball was the only exception to this rule, and thankfully, the shorts were just long enough to cover most of my legs. Even then, I felt uncomfortable wearing them.

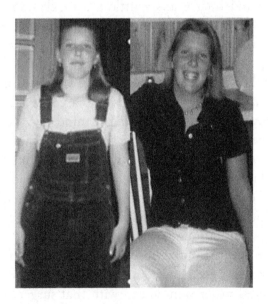

(left) Me in grade 8 hiding under overalls, pulling back my cowlick, and concealing my "gummy" smile.

(right) Me at age 15 with a fake smile and the weight of self-hatred on my shoulders. This was just before my mom's life-altering career change.

At the start of high-school, I had a falling out with my main group of friends, which left me in a brand-new school feeling very lonely and even worse about myself than I already did. I still don't remember what happened or why, but this fall-out was the catalyst of many challenges for me. I started getting bullied on the school bus, which only contributed to my enormous pile of self-hatred and poor self-esteem. I couldn't always avoid the bus, but when I could, I would walk home from school, which was at least a twenty-five-minute walk across town. I'm not certain why I internalized the hurt I experienced from all of this, but I did. I started hating myself more than ever.

I quickly began to think and even believe there was something wrong with me. That somehow everyone else was normal, and I wasn't. I wasn't pretty, I wasn't good enough, and I wasn't like everyone else. I often turned to alcohol on the weekends as a means to cope with the way I felt about myself. It made me feel better for a while and allowed me to escape.

One night at a party, I combined way too much booze with a lot of marijuana and almost went over the edge. I don't remember all of the details, but I do remember that a fight with a friend landed me in the bathroom, and it was there that I took all of the anger, hatred, and frustration I was feeling out on myself. I broke a beer bottle and cut my wrist with its jagged edge.

To this day, I don't have a solid answer as to why I cut myself. All I know for sure is that, as it bled, I looked down in fear, horror, and extreme shame at what I had done to myself. I immediately regretted it. I knew within seconds that it was wrong, and I wanted to take it back. *How could I have been so stupid*, was the question I beat myself up with just moments after. As I sobered up, I felt increasingly worse. I was embarrassed and ashamed.

The cut was not quite deep enough to actually cause me harm but it came way too close. I'm certain it wasn't that I even wanted to die. I think maybe instead I wanted someone to care. I wanted the bullying to stop. I wanted to fit in and feel like I belonged. I wanted to feel loved by others. Truthfully, though, and most of all, I wanted to love myself.

At the time, the consequences of my actions weren't really a thought in my mind. I wasn't thinking at all. I was reacting to how I felt in that moment. I knew I disliked myself and my body. I knew I felt lonely and rejected by my friends, and I felt as if there was something flawed about me. I knew I was angry and frustrated with myself and my life, but what I didn't know was something extremely important.

What I didn't know was that everyone feels this way sometimes, especially teenagers, and especially those who are bullied. The feelings I was having were, and are, completely normal human, but they were feelings I hadn't learned to cope with. Learning to talk openly about what we're feeling and going through is what can help us all deal with the many struggles of life.

Why do we hide our sorrows and flaunt our happiness? Why do so many people, moms included, suffer in silence? Too many moms have postpartum depression, exhaustion, anxiety, and are feeling overwhelmed and defeated. What's worse is that we've created a culture where they feel too ashamed even to admit it, let alone ask for help. The expectation is that a mom can do it all and more, without ever needing to ask for help. As a result, so many moms keep going until they crash.

Doing what I did was not stupid, as I once had thought. I know that now. It was a sign that I needed help, support, compassion, and love. It was a sign that I needed to learn how to cope with the feelings I was having rather than resorting to drugs and alcohol to numb them. The great news is that it was not too late to learn all of this. Thankfully.

That night, Graham came to my rescue. What I remember most was that he didn't judge me. He listened, he cared, and for the first time, I felt genuinely loved by someone other than my family. This began a friendship that soon led to true love. A love that I am grateful for every single day.

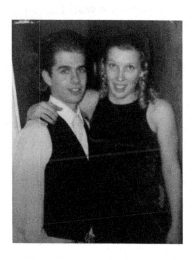

Graham and I are high school sweet hearts. This is us at our semi-formal.

For years afterward, I felt ashamed of what I had done. So much so that I worked to hide the marks on my wrist and bury the story with my silence. I never told a single person what had happened. I feared their judgements. I worried they would think I was crazy and avoid getting to know me because of it. I cared too much what others thought and never cared enough for myself. A lot has changed.

As I wrote this book, I debated not including this part of my story, but I felt it was important. Maybe it can help prevent a similar story from ever happening to someone else. Maybe it can console someone who is feeling the way that I did. Sadly, there are many people in our world struggling. Too many are turning to drugs and alcohol to cope. Too many are hating themselves, feeling hopeless, and, sadly, even contemplating ending their life. Suicide is devastating, and it's sweeping through our world at an alarming rate. I'm prepared to be brave enough to start the conversation and honest enough to share with you that I could have easily been one of these victims. If I can help one mother or son or daughter or friend realize the best years are ahead of them, it's worth the world knowing my whole story. Suicide doesn't just kill the pain from the present and past, it kills the entire future, and I'm so thankful it didn't kill mine.

A few nights ago Zachary woke me up at 4 am asking for snuggles. He's two so it sounded more like "nuggle mama?" As I lay in bed with him cozied into my arms and a heart filled with love for him I thought, *wow, I would have missed this moment.* I've had thousands of moments like this one that I would have missed.

What I can tell you now is that I am free from that shame I once felt so deeply. The scar that covers over all that pain is a daily reminder to me that life is fragile. It makes me thankful for the gift of every single day. It reminds me that I am loved, I am special, I am beautiful, and I am enough. It has taught me that much like scar tissue in comparison to regular skin, I too am stronger than I used to be. Wounds heal, and people can too when given the love and support they need. I'm living proof. Now I have a passion to teach others just how dangerous self-hatred can be.

I am thankful that I am still here. The years since then have been the best years of my life. I cannot imagine having missed out on the amazing opportunity to know and love my three boys. Had things gone differently back then, I would have missed out on so much. I would have never had the chance to be a mom, to be loved by Graham, to help inspire change in other's lives in such an amazing way, or to experience all of the wonderful things that my future has to offer. I believe God has a plan for everyone's life, and today I am blessed to be living that plan for my own. I do not take a single day for granted. Every day, I am thankful that cut wasn't quite deep enough.

Whatever your struggle, you deserve to live, and I promise the future can be better. Pain is temporary. Dark places do not have to last. Know that you are loved, worthy, special, important, and that you offer something no one else can. The world is a better place because you are in it. It's important you begin to discover how truly amazing you are and stop believing anything to the contrary. It's time to start loving yourself.

It's also important you share your feelings with others. People can only help if they know what you're going through. For all of the talking us moms do, we really do need to talk more about what really matters. Chances are good you are not the only one feeling the way you feel: overwhelmed, tired, stressed, frustrated, and lonely. Sharing your struggles is liberating for yourself and for others. Hiding them and putting on a picture-perfect, life-is-rosy false face only isolates you and keeps those around you isolated as well. Trust me, your loved ones want to help, and fellow moms want to hear how you're really feeling because it will allow them to share the truth about how they are feeling, too. Life is hard. Being a mom is darn hard. If we can be open about our struggles, we can set a whole lot of people free from theirs.

For me, being fifteen years old and facing all of this mostly alone was not easy. The light after this very dark time came when my mother began making some changes in our home that would change me forever. *Did I mention that moms are powerful and the impact they can have is incredible?* She introduced healthier foods and supplements like vitamins and minerals. Because she was experiencing some health challenges, she began exploring natural options to get better. After many courses and a much healthier way of eating, her health was restored, and her career path permanently altered.

When I was sixteen, my mom took a massive leap of faith. She went from a registered nurse of thirty years to an owner and operator of a natural health clinic and fitness center called Health Options. She quit her job because she felt she was only seeing people get worse rather than better. She wanted to work in the preventative health field where she could help people live healthier and prevent disease before it occurred. This became the catalyst that changed my life!

I started working at the front desk of my mothers gym. I also started exercising regularly. I lifted weights and attended cardio classes and learned more about healthy eating and proper supplementation. In less than a year, I lost all of the extra weight and was looking and feeling healthier on the outside. I was leaner and stronger and learning to fuel my body well. That being said, a healthy outside begins on the inside, and the inside of me still needed a lot of work. I had the order mixed up.

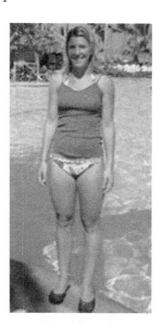

After losing the weight but before learning to love myself.

Losing weight is a physical and a mental process. Your body may lose the weight, but your mind needs to lose it as well. This takes a lot of work and a lot of time. The challenge for me was that I was still the same, insecure, self-deprecating person on the inside. I was not in love with myself and my body even though it had changed. I carried all of my inadequacies and insecurities with me into this new body I sported.

As I became more educated within the fitness world and started working as a personal trainer and nutrition consultant, I began wanting to look the part. I wanted a six pack because I believed all trainers should have that. I wanted more muscle and less body fat. Most of all, I wanted slimmer legs, even though they already were slim, my mind just hadn't caught up with the weight loss. I still had it out for my legs.

This is the problem with so many weight loss programs out there and, in many cases, with the fitness and weight loss industry as a whole. They don't address the mind. Instead, the focus is solely on the body and making it smaller and leaner. Working on the mental side of weight loss is the key to sustaining lifelong changes. Your mind must come on the journey, too. In fact, without it, the physical changes usually do not last.

Even though I had physically re-shaped my body, I had not changed my poor self-talk. I had not worked on loving myself exactly as I was. In fact, most of what I was doing was coming from a place of hating my body rather than loving it. This lack of awareness of needing to work on the inside me left doors of insecurities open, and I began to think I needed to do drastic things to look and be fit.

I restricted my food intake, I lived on a diet, I over-exercised, and I jumped into fitness competitions to make my body comply to the ideals of what I thought it should look like. If I was going to be a fitness professional, I was darn well going to look like one, too.

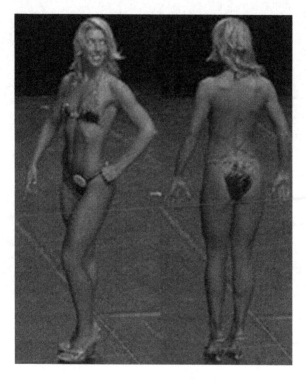

My first of several fitness competitions.

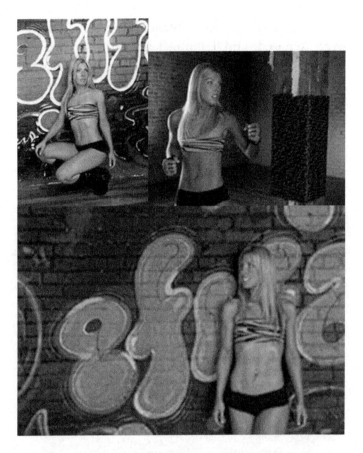

Photo shoot before learning to LOVE my body.
Despite looking great, I didn't think I looked great
at all.

One fitness competition turned into years of
competing and getting into a world of photo shoots,
fitness modeling, sponsorships, and endless dieting
down and exercising to be lean. Though my body
finally looked the part, believe it or not, I was still not

loving my appearance. I would get up on stage and be compared to other girls and judges would make subjective decisions about who should win and who shouldn't.

Despite doing better at each competition, judges notes would come back that my legs needed work and were too big, that my waist was thick, and that I lacked confidence. The confidence part was true; I never felt good enough. I needed to deal with all of those issues I had accumulated in the past before I could ever move forward with confidence and self-love.

The judges feedback fed my insecurities even more. I would walk away from a competition feeling worse about myself than when I had started. I was spiraling into a scary cycle of dieting, over-exercising, and prancing on stage to be compared and rated based on my appearance.

Don't get me wrong, these types of competitions require intense discipline, dedication, athleticism, and darn hard work. I am not at all negating that. Many who enter them walk away completely unaffected by judges notes or the process of comparing to determine the winner. I wish that were me. Unfortunately, I walked away feeling worse about myself rather than better. I needed to get healthy on the inside.

Graham, who had been my husband for a few years at this point, was getting increasingly worried about me and kept asking me why I wanted to do this competition thing. Because of his background in sports psychology, I knew he was digging for more than a simple, surface-level answer. He always has excellent questions that get me thinking deeper. This time, though, much like others, I could not give him a solid answer. All I knew for sure was that I was on a mission to look good and to me that meant ripped and lean and like a photoshopped picture on the cover of a fitness magazine.

Just after what would be my last competition ever, a pivotal moment changed so many things for me. My sister Tricia invited me to come and watch her triathlon. She had been training for it for several months, and I was excited to go and support her at the finish line. She had supported me on stage, and I was thankful for the opportunity to return this love. I knew she had worked hard for this event and couldn't wait to cheer her across the finish line of a 750-metre swim, 30-kilometre bike ride, and 5-kilometre run.

Seeing her finish the triathlon was life-altering for me. What I noticed about her was that she was completely consumed by pure happiness. That finish line made her proud of what her body was able to do. What I also noticed was that her focus was not on caring what she looked like, instead it was about caring how her body had performed. She celebrated her strength, determination, and perseverance. Her hair was a mess, and she was covered in sweat, but none of that mattered. She was so proud and happy with herself, and we all felt the same way for her.

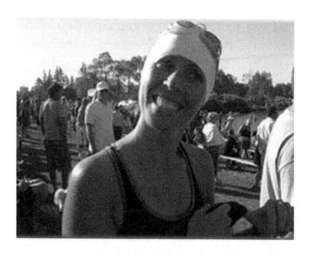

My sister Tricia smiling big at the triathlon that changed so much for me.

The triathlon reminded me of a dream that had been hiding in my heart for many years. I loved to run and had always wanted to run a marathon. I had set running aside while training for fitness competitions because I wanted to focus my efforts on that, but after Tricia's event, I was ready to re-visit my dream.

Realizing that whenever I finished a competition I felt down on myself, not good enough, and very unhappy with my body was one of the best things that could have ever happened. It was then that I knew fitness competing was not for me. I needed a change that would take the focus off of looks and give me the empowerment that came with crossing a finish line. It was time to train for that marathon, and Graham was fully on board to support me. I speculate he was very relieved that I had seen the light.

Just like that, I set my competing days aside and began to run. Not because I wanted to see how many calories I was burning or because I wanted to look a certain way, but because it made me happy and gave me a sense of pride in what my body could do. What a switch!

I took several sports nutrition courses to learn more about the importance of fueling my body for an event like this one. I knew how to lean down for stage day, but I didn't know how to fuel up for race day, and trust me, these are two very different things.

What I learned was that I needed to fuel my body rather than deprive it. If my body was going to carry me 42.2 kilometres and perform all of the training leading up to that, it needed good fuel and a lot more of it. My days of living on a carefully portioned eating regime were over. Taking these chains off was freeing, and the best part was that somewhere in the process of logging kilometres, I began to heal from self-hatred. I fell in love with what my body was capable of doing. My self-talk became more positive. My focus became on what I was able to do rather than on what I was lacking, and for the first time ever, I actually felt good about myself and my body.

With each run, I felt a sense of pride I had honestly never felt before in my entire life. Crossing the finish line of that marathon was quite literally life-altering. The confidence I gained from running ignited a passion for athleticism and exploring all of the amazing things that my body could do when given the love that it truly deserved.

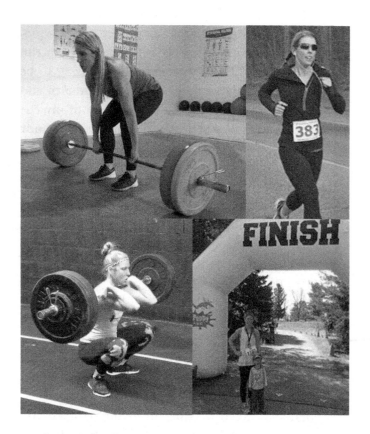

I continued to run and still do. I've completed countless races and then added duathlons to my list of challenges along with Olympic lifting. Nothing builds confidence for me like being able to run and bike fast, lift heavy things, and train and prepare for events that challenge my body and my mind.

Bringing this new viewpoint to my clients has been life-changing for them, too. I've become a much better coach who does not primarily focus her client's minds on the importance of how they look. Instead, it's about how they feel, how they perform, and what their bodies can do. We celebrate non-scale victories. Being able to do a pushup, lift a heavy weight, or run for a kilometer without stopping is something to be proud of. It's so awesome to see the confidence and sense of empowerment that grows in each of my clients as they learn how strong and amazing their body actually is.

Despite countless stage fitness competitions, photo shoots, sponsorships, and placing well, I always came away feeling not good enough, defeated, and disappointed by how my body looked. Fast forward to countless races and lifting events and I always come away feeling proud of myself and so appreciative of what my body can do.

This switch from disliking my body for what it was not, to loving it for all that it is has been amazing, to say the least. I went from exercising and eating a certain way because I hated my body, to exercising and eating a certain way because I loved and appreciated it.

There's so much freedom in loving yourself and your body. It's not conceited, it's liberating. It's not prideful, it's peaceful. You only get one body; it's time to embrace and accept it exactly as it is. Why spend one more day out of love with your actual life-long home?

Show love to your body with healthy fuel, regular exercise, rest, stretching, and, above all, gratitude for the amazing work of art that it is and all that it does for you. Your body was perfectly designed and wonderfully made, and it deserves your love and acceptance.

Look in the mirror and embrace all of your unique and beautiful imperfections. You are special, valuable, significant, and amazing, and it's time to start knowing it. Life is far too short to waste another second unhappy with who you are or how you look. You deserve to be confident and happy and at peace with your incredible self.

I completely understand being unhappy about stretch marks, scars, wrinkles, loose skin, cellulite, and excess fat, but if you can't change it, it's time to come to terms with it. My scar from a bad decision is now a part of me and my story. Every stretch mark I have is also a part of me. The loose skin around my belly from having babies is also a part of me. I can't change these things, so I have come to a place of embracing them. I refuse to hate them, be ashamed of them, or ever cover them up. I was beautiful before them, and I am beautiful with them. So are you.

Over time, I've come to realize that my self-loathing was never caused by a fitness competition. It was worsened by them, but I caused it by neglecting my mind. I didn't go back to that insecure, self-hating little girl and tell her she was beautiful. I didn't work on my inside, so even though the outside looked healthy and strong, the inside was the opposite of that.

Racing, lifting, and competing as an athlete did not cause me to love myself, but they did assist in giving me the confidence I needed to do that mind work. Now that I have, I am a whole new me. It may sound cheesy, but it's true. It's one reason my husband and I called our business New U. When you begin to love yourself, you really do become new.

Today, I love me. I love the cowlick that makes my bangless hair sweep up and over my forehead. I love the bump on my nose that adds distinction and character to my face. I love my gummy smile that is beautiful and unique, and now that I see that same smile on my children's precious faces, I think I love it even more. I love the muscles I have worked so hard to have. I love the amazingly strong and fast legs that have carried me over countless finish lines, lifted very heavy weights, and won many medals. I love what my body and mind can do when given the right fuel and the right training and, above all, the right amount of love.

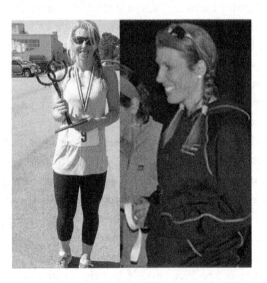

1st place overall in a 5k road race, 3rd place overall in an 8k road race.

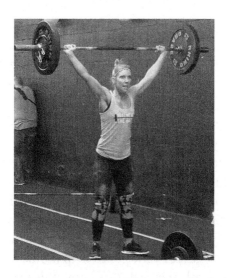

Me at a lifting competition. My team finished 2nd place in our category.

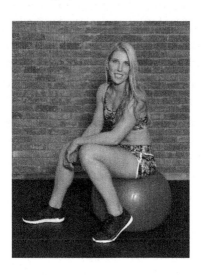

I am confident, happier, content with who I am, and totally liberated from the cycle of disliking myself and my body. I realize now that all of my challenges and struggles can be used to help liberate others from theirs. I have a skill and a passion for motivating and inspiring others, and I am so thankful to be here still to be able to do just that. I've worked hard at better self-talk and self-care, and over time, I have stopped beating myself up, stopped feeling guilty, stopped calling myself horrible names, and stopped picking at my uniqueness. Instead, I embrace everything that makes me who I am.

Coming to a place of being at peace with myself is an incredible feeling too good to keep for myself. It's completely freeing, and there really is no better way to live. I love that I now get to help moms everywhere fall in love with themselves. I know this is not an easy process, but I also know it's totally worth the effort. I want you to be liberated for the rest of your life, and that starts with doing some mind work.

Again, this is not an overnight switch, but there are things that you can do to get to a place of being thankful for and appreciating yourself and your body and all that you are.

The first step is awareness. Being aware of your self-talk will enable you to begin to change it. Every time you find yourself trying on clothes or looking in the mirror or at a picture of yourself, be aware of your thoughts. Then, immediately correct them. Do not entertain the negative ones or give them a chance to grow or fester; slap them in the face instead. Sometimes, you'll need to be loud.

We cannot think and speak at the same time. Speaking a positive affirmation aloud will hijack your brains thoughts. Immediately, you will have to stop thinking what you were thinking in order to speak.

The next time the thought that you are ugly crosses your mind, speak aloud, "I am beautiful!" The next time you think that you are a failure, a bad mom, a disappointment, or whatever else your mind attempts to say to you, speak aloud, "I am doing my best; I am a work in progress; I am amazing." Making an "I am" list like the bookmark I've provided you within this book is powerful. Speaking it aloud is even more powerful.

When your children hear you speak these kind words about yourself, they learn how to speak kind words about themselves, too. This is a skill I wish more adults had learned as children, myself included. It would have saved me years of grief. You hold the power to break the self-loathing cycle and show your children how to love themselves first. Imagine what life would be like for them if they never had to go through it disliking themselves or their bodies. That's absolute freedom!

Awareness and brain hijacks take practice and time. Daily affirmations without action usually do not make much of a difference. Action will be necessary for you to get the changes you are hoping for. Change takes time and practice. Gratitude is one key to changing the way you view yourself. Maybe your legs are not your favorite feature. Write a list of all of the things you are thankful they can do. Maybe you have some insecurities about your smile or your nose. Write a list of all of the things you appreciate about your smile and your nose. Make a list and then review it daily.

You cannot be grateful and hateful at the same time; it's neurologically impossible. In fact, this works for a world of things. You cannot be stressed, sad, lonely, angry, frustrated, or have anxiety and be grateful at the same time. Next time your self-talk isn't good, or your children are stressing you out, or you are experiencing fear or anger, try starting a list of all of the things you are grateful for and watch the magic happen.

This works very well on airplanes. I hate flying—or I should say, I used to hate it. I would get anxious and stressed even a few days before boarding. It's one reason my husband and I have not done a lot of traveling.

It had been almost seven years since we had been on a kid-free vacation, and it was long overdue. I agreed to go and was thankful for the opportunity to take the trip and for having childcare help, but I was dreading the flights. This time was much different, though. This time I practiced gratitude. I made a long list of all of the things I was grateful for while I was on the plane, and as we flew, whenever I felt anxious, I would read over my list and add to it.

Guess what? I actually fell asleep during the flight, in the middle of the day. Sure, I had to fight some negative thoughts and work hard to steer my mind toward gratitude and not fear, but once I did, I was stress-free, and I could actually sleep. You can do it, too.

Another thing you can do that is very effective in reprogramming your self-talk is to get a picture of yourself when you were a child. Set it as your background on your phone or your computer. Hang it somewhere in your home where you will see it often. When your self-talk is negative, look at that beautiful face and ask yourself, *Would I tell her that?* Reminding ourselves of that precious, fragile child within us is a powerful tool for changing the way we speak to ourselves.

There are a few things I want you to know, and they are true whether you believe them to be at this moment or not. You are beautiful, exactly as you are. You are not too big, too small, too weak, too loud, too quiet, too weird, or too anything. You are just right exactly as you are. You are capable, even on the days you don't feel you are. Being a mom can make you feel completely incapable, but if you choose to, it can also make you feel like the superhero you actually are. You really do have a choice.

You are worthy of being loved by others and yourself. You are important and special, and you matter. I also hope you can come to a place in your life, as I have in mine, where you can let go of all of the negative comments and mean self-talk from loved ones and strangers and begin to love yourself, this very moment, exactly as you are. You deserve that love more than anything in the whole world.

If you want your children to learn to be kind to themselves, you need to lead the way. The power to liberate them and you is between your own two ears. Guard your mind. Do not allow negativity to enter it. Use your mouth as a weapon to combat all negative thoughts that try to enter. Speak positive, healthy words about yourself to yourself—aloud—so your mind can hear your voice.

Last, always remember this, loving yourself is the very best medicine. It cures a world of ailments, so please dose daily. Doing so will change how you feel about yourself, and that has the power to impact many areas of your life. The reward is that the rest of your life will be filled with harmony between you and the only body you will ever have.

Action Items

Awareness. It's time to pay attention to your thoughts more than you ever have. What are you saying to yourself daily? When was the last time you thought, *Wow I'm an excellent mother* (you are) or *My body is amazing!* (it really is). It's time to start thinking like this much more often. First, bring awareness to your self-talk, then work to correct all of the lies.

Positive affirmations. You may need to combat that negative movie reel in your head with positive words spoken aloud. Some days will be easy, some days won't. Whether easy or difficult, keep speaking good and healthy words about yourself. The next time you think to yourself that you look ugly or fat, say aloud, "This outfit is lucky to have me in it. I am beautiful inside and out." Fight back!

Gratitude. Be thankful for all your body can do, for the opportunity to be a mother, and for each and every new day you get. Write out a list of everything you are thankful for, and please include your amazing arms that lift your beautiful children and your incredible body that helped grow them.

Compile an "I Am" list. This is something I regularly have my clients do. What you place after the words "I am" are incredibly powerful. Start with a list of 3 to 5 and work your way up to a list of 100. For example, I am strong, capable, smart, and worthy. Read this list when you're feeling defeated, unhappy, lonely, or are having a difficult day.

Change your focus. It's perfectly healthy to have a weight-loss goal, but remember you'll need to tackle that goal from a place of loving your body rather than disliking it. Because you love your body, you will do what is necessary to lose the unhealthy weight. Changing your focus can also mean making a shift from a looks-centered goal to a performance-based goal. Learn what your body is capable of by signing up for a 5k run, obstacle event, or bike race.

Let go. Forgive all those people who have made negative comments about you and your body and remember, part of forgiving is forgetting. There is massive liberation in letting go. Moms carry enough stuff as it is. Lighten the load by letting go of all of the unimportant things and holding tight to what matters most.

4

Switch # 3– The Food Switch

When it comes to food, moms deserve gourmet meals and uninterrupted time to sit down and enjoy them. They deserve personal chefs who have healthy food prepared in advance so all they have to do is show up, sit down, and eat. Moms take care of everyone else, and I genuinely feel they deserve to have someone taking care of them in the same way. (I know, I know. In the words of my father, "You're a dreamer, Al." He's right, but a mom can dream, can't she?)

Unfortunately, life with kids and life in general is far from conducive to this kind of luxury for most people. If you're one of the lucky moms, you may get the opportunity to enjoy a delicious pampered meal a few times a year or at least once a year on Mother's Day. This year, I was given breakfast in bed, most of which was stolen from me by my very hungry Zachary. Of course, it's the thought that counts, and I love that they made an effort to make me feel special.

The reality is that no one is going to do it all for you. In fact, chances are good that the opposite is true—you are the one doing it all for everyone else. This is why it's imperative you make the switch to making yourself a priority and loving yourself first. Then you'll see the value and importance of taking time to fuel your body with healthy food because you'll love yourself enough to do just that.

I have a few effective guidelines for you to live by that will transform your body and your health and keep you looking and feeling your best for the rest of your life. Trust me, they work. They are easy to implement, do not require too much of your time or energy, and they will get you and your children on track to a healthy relationship with food. Before I get into that, there are a few food switches that must be made by all moms—forever.

First, no more toddler leftovers. A lot of busy moms are living off of leftover food. You may be one of them, or you may know one of them. It's very common, and I totally understand why it happens, but it has to stop. Because many moms are in survival mode and catering to every call (there's that self-sacrificial lie again), they are not always taking the time to prepare food for themselves. Instead, they are fueling up with coffee and living off the scraps their little ones leave behind.

Sometimes they will sit down and enjoy a snack or meal with the kids, but most moms are focusing on their to-do list while their kids eat. Then, as they clean up plates from snack time, they eat the remains—a few, fast half-eaten strawberries or crackers, maybe some cucumber and the remnants of a sandwich—and then quickly move on to the next thing on the list of a million things to do. I know because I've done it, too, and I work with so many moms who have also done it. By the end of the day, they may get a decent dinner, but sometimes even that is compromised by a rush to afterschool activities.

The kids always get fed, but moms will go for hours on empty. By sleep time, when they finally stop and get a few quiet minutes kid-free, they are hungry. Tired and hungry leaves people reaching for unhealthy options. The chances of having a spinach salad at 9:00 p.m. are pretty slim. Sugary, carbohydrate-dense calories washed down by some (or a lot of) wine ends their day.

If you're a working mom, life could look a little different. You may grab something fast on your way to work and wolf it down on the way. You may get a sit-down lunch and then come home to a fast-paced evening of picking kids up, preparing dinner, cleaning, driving to sporting events, and then preparing for it all over again tomorrow. Comfort foods and wine are the common go-to at the end of a long day for most moms. If this is you, you're not alone, and I'm here to help.

I reserve all judgement because I really do get it. I've been a stay-at-home mom and a working mom. I also promise that I have a better way. It starts with you making the switch that you will never again settle for less than you deserve. Though I do mean no more toddler leftovers in the literal sense, I also mean that from now on you get a healthy breakfast, lunch, dinner, and snacks. You make the time to sit down and enjoy them because you deserve the best and because you are the mom and you need all of the energy you can get.

You would never let your child go hungry, you would never have them miss a meal, and I bet you always try your best to make sure they get something healthy to eat most of the time. Why on earth are you not held to this same standard? You prepare amazing meals and snacks for your little ones, and they sit down and are given the time to enjoy them. It's time to do the same for yourself because you're worth it.

Part of that "mom tired" I spoke about earlier comes with being under-fueled or fueled by unhealthy quick energy foods. It's time to give your body the fuel it needs so it can give you the energy you need because, as I already said, and I know you'll agree, you need energy.

We don't expect our cars to run on empty. They can't. It's time to stop expecting your body to run on empty. We don't expect our cars to perform well on crappy, cheap gas. Again, they can't. It's time to stop expecting your body to function on unhealthy, crappy foods.

I'm not telling you that you need to be perfect all of the time. Trust me, I am far from that. It's much more about progress than it is about perfection. (We'll chat about that a little later.) Your body needs healthy food to be at its best. It's time to stop settling for anything less. Food is fuel. Fill up often, and fill up on the best quality, not the scraps. Eat the way you wish to feel. As cheesy as it may sound (pardon the food pun), it really is true. If you want to feel good, you need to fuel good. This is easier said than done, but again, I am here to help.

Now, can I open up the can of dieting worms? Let's talk for a few minutes about diets. This dirty word doesn't deserve much of our time, but I need to tell you the second food switch, and that is never to diet again.

You now know that I've been there, done that, and thankfully learned from it. For two full years, I lived in a world of food restriction, calorie calculating, macronutrient counting, and fitness competing. For two years, I lived on a diet, and trust me, this is no way to live. Dieting is for crazy people, and it will make you crazy if you weren't before you started. I can't imagine life without chocolate covered almonds or salt and vinegar chips, and I'm very thankful that these things will never be off limits to me again. I don't have to earn them (I'm not a dog, and neither are you), and I especially don't have to feel bad about eating them.

To get my muscles to show for photoshoots and stage day, I would become more and more depleted of essential nutrients, nutrients necessary for proper health. Despite looking the complete picture of health and strength on the big day, I was dehydrated and hungry, not to mention over-exercised and exhausted. I was mentally tired of always saying no to certain foods, of always thinking about my next meal, missing out on the birthday cake at birthday dinners, and choosing salads over pumpkin pie on Thanksgiving. I wanted the pumpkin pie, too.

I thought that I needed to eat this way and live restricted if I was going to look thin and lean. I was very wrong. You do not have to diet to lose weight. Remember that I mentioned becoming more educated about food? As soon as I learned the power that food has to increase our energy levels, decrease our body fat, and improve our performance, my entire way of eating changed and so did my body.

I stopped dieting and restricting, and my body became stronger, healthier, and leaner. I started eating quality carbohydrates and more healthy fats and proteins, and suddenly I was lean without having to do hours of cardio or live on a diet. I found a balance that allows me to enjoy a glass of wine or pumpkin pie or birthday cake and does not interfere with my goals or my health. I can't wait to share my tips with you. You'll love the results you get, how great you begin to feel, and above all, how freeing it is never to diet again.

There is a balance you must find to live healthily and make a lifestyle change for you and your family. It starts with vowing to never diet or live on any type of food restriction program again. I've worked with thousands of woman over the years who have dieted to the point of causing metabolic syndrome, nutrient deficiencies, thyroid problems, poor self-esteem, and much more. It's not worth it, and it's not healthy.

Not only do diets and restricting food groups or food intake not work and can leave you physically unhealthy, they also leave you feeling defeated and hopeless. Most people gain all of the weight back and more. Along with this comes a cycle of on again off again. The yo-yo life is a horrible recipe for an unhealthy body and mind.

Counting, calculating, weighing, cutting, totaling, restricting, starting again on Monday, and the guilt that comes along with unhealthy food choices, all must stop now. I find this to be the most difficult switch for many to make because we've been programmed to being on something and used to falling off of it.

We've also been programmed to have a tremendous amount of emotion, mainly guilt, surrounding our food choices. You have to break and change your mindset about food to move forward toward a healthy relationship with it. Not only will this help you, but it will help your kids, too.

Children who see a mom yo-yo are much more likely to yo-yo themselves. Work at making healthy eating a lifestyle rather than something you start and stop. This will establish a consistently healthy relationship with food, and as a result, will send a clear and healthy message to your children.

When I tell clients, they will never fall off of anything again because they are no longer on anything, they usually feel a massive and immediate sense of relief. They also often experience a bit of confusion trying to sort what that looks like. Trust me, I get it. The world tells us the best way to lose weight is to diet, and the next diet trend comes out looking enticing and convincing with all of its science and glitz, and now I am telling you to jump off the diet wagon and never stress about your next bite again. Stay with me, and I promise it will be worth it.

One amazing mom I know started our program with a conversation that went like this: "I understand that I'm not on a diet, but could you just give me a total calorie count that I am allowed to have in a day so I know what and how much to eat?"

My response? "No, I can't because that would be a diet, and we don't do diets! What I can give you are some amazing guidelines to follow that will help you learn how to eat healthy, off of a diet, for the rest of your life."

She gave me a blank stare and then a few seconds later started to cry. For years, she had been in the diet cycle desperately trying to lose weight and feel better and that day was the day the cycle broke. The emotional release was the beginning of a lot of amazing healing.

Though it, of course, took some adjusting to, and a lot of mental and physical work on her part, she made the switch and rarely stresses about food anymore. Her children are also learning how to fuel their bodies with healthy choices. The whole family is benefiting. Talk about liberation! The freedom that comes when you can stop dieting and, as they say, start living, is honestly life and body changing. Plus, the trickle-down effect on your children is worth it.

I've said it before—your children will be what they see. I know you have good intentions, but if they see a mom who is constantly yo-yoing and always on a diet, these actions speak louder than any of your words. If they see that Mom is always eating salads or tiny restricted portions, they may get the message that "this is how moms should eat" and even internalize it to become "this is how I should eat, too." If they see that mom is always avoiding carbs, always nixing fat or popping diet pills, and always weighing in, they will get the wrong message about healthy eating and living. I know that's not what you want for your kids. Me, either!

Seeing this modeled creates a lot of confusion about food even though this is not your intention. It has to stop for their sake and for your sake. Stop now before they begin to shape their beliefs around nutrition and healthy eating and body image. You may not think they notice, but I promise you they do.

Your child is always watching. The messages you send about food will become the foundation of what healthy living is for them, for the rest of their life. Choose your messaging wisely. Make your actions speak by modeling a healthy relationship with food from this moment on.

If you have older children, it's not too late. Remember, I was fifteen when my mom made that healthy switch in our home, and it was one of the best things that ever happened to me. Whatever their age, when you make the food switch, they will move forward in their own life with complete and total freedom surrounding food and trust me, it's the best way to live.

Now that you know the nutrition switches to work on, let's talk about the easiest way to transform your body and your health with food. I've listed the guidelines that I follow, my coaching team follows, and all of our clients live by. Not only are they effective for weight loss, increasing energy, improving overall health, and getting you great results, but they are also simple to implement into your daily routine. From now on there will be no more stress about food ever again.

Gone are the days of calorie totals, macro counting, and meal plans. I used to do these for my clients and spend hours calculating to make sure they were done just right. The truth is that every single body thrives off of these ten simple guidelines, so why live any other way?

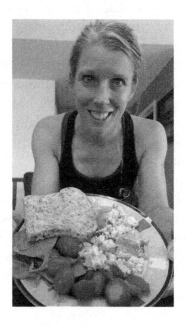

1. **Hydrate often.** To stay energized, decrease body fat, increase fat storage utilization, minimize water retention, back pain, headaches, and a world of other ailments—drink water! Aim for eight to ten glasses a day. Your urine should be

light yellow to almost clear all day long. Water is what you're made of, so water is what your body needs most. Drink up.

2. **Eat green to stay lean.** As you know, all vegetables are excellent for your health. Most people do not consume enough of them. It's important you eat the rainbow of veggies to ensure you get everything your body needs to stay healthy. We encourage our moms to consume veggies at least three times a day.

   Green veggies bring with them a world of nutrients into your body and help it stay strong and lean. Aim to increase your green veggie intake by throwing spinach or asparagus into your eggs, having a green smoothie with kale or spinach or arugula added, eating salads, raw veggies with hummus, stir-fries, soups, wraps, and having steamed greens with your dinner (broccoli, asparagus, green beans, brussels sprouts, etc.). When you eat more greens, you will get leaner, and most importantly, healthier. You'll also be getting more nutrients into your body, which will leave you feeling much more energized.

3. **Eat four to five times a day.** Kids really do have this one figured out. Obviously, too much snacking or worse, grazing, is not ideal for weight loss but not enough eating isn't either. I give my clients a range of eating four to five times a day. Rather than grazing all day long, try to organize your day to have set meal and snack times. For example, my day looks like this: breakfast, lunch, snack, supper, and another snack if needed. If

you're not hungry for a fifth meal, don't have it. If you are, then do (more on hunger distinction soon).

4. **Combine your macronutrients.** Eat a protein (roughly palm size), carbohydrate (roughly fist size), and fat (roughly thumb size) at every meal. Combining macronutrients ensures you get enough protein and a healthy amount of carbohydrates and fats. These macronutrients are essential for your health. Look and feel your best all day long by pairing these together at every meal.

   You've no doubt witnessed a child with low blood sugar a time or two? Silly question, of course you have. Well, guess what? Adults can be just as moody. Combining macronutrients regulates blood sugar levels keeping your mood and energy levels stable all day. It also minimizes cravings and is great for fat loss and fat storage utilization, and it keeps you feeling satisfied longer.

   Combining your macronutrients will give your body the energy it needs to feel and perform at its best. From now on, don't have a piece of fruit on its own. Add a protein and some healthy fat to keep blood glucose levels in check and trust me you really will feel the difference.

5. **Consume food roughly every three to four hours.** The hunger window is different for every person, but generally, after a properly portioned meal, your body can go roughly three to four hours without needing another meal. It's not

necessary to eat between meals. Leaving this time gap allows your body to use its stored fat as fuel.

Remember, you are not "on" anything, so this can be made to work for you and your life. This isn't about being rigid, it's simply a guideline. For example, some days you may eat every three hours and feel satisfied, other days because of schedules and life maybe it's three and a half or four hours. Either way, stick to the gaps as best you can and remember that it doesn't have to be perfect to be progress.

6. **Replenish your gut flora daily.** Without a large and diverse microbiome (bacteria in your gut), your entire body will be compromised, including your immune system, but also your digestive system, and definitely your ability to metabolize body fat. Incorporate more fermented foods and drinks into your daily eating regime, supplement with a quality probiotic, and limit the amount of sugar, refined foods, medications, and environmental toxins that you are exposed to. These can decrease your gut flora and cause imbalances. To increase your healthy gut flora, be sure to eat fruits and veggies and nuts and seeds, along with garlic and onions, as these foods (and many others) are prebiotics (food for the good bacteria) that will help your gut stay healthy.

7. **Consume a variety of foods.** Variety is an important part of eating healthy. Your body requires a diversified menu to get the many different nutrients that it needs. Trying new fruits, veggies, and other foods as often as you can is

very important. Rather than getting stuck in a routine of the same old foods, day in and day out, cook something different for dinner once in a while. This does not have to be overwhelming. Bring one new food home each time you go grocery shopping. Get your kids involved in tasting and enjoy the fun of exploring new things together.

8. **Live with balance, not restriction.** Great news— not being on a diet means that you can have that glass of wine or favorite snack once in a while. You should also enjoy birthday cake and ice cream with your children, and by all means, go out with your girlfriends or husband and order your favorite meal or dessert. Just don't do it every day, and do not feel bad about it for even one second. Strive to choose healthy most of the time, and do your best not to over-eat.

This healthy lifestyle switch is all about balance. It's about eating healthy and making healthful choices most of the time and allowing yourself to have a few extras once in a while. Just as you don't allow your children to live off of sugar (we both know how that would go), you should not live off of unhealthy options, either. Do your best to eat well, and once in a while, allow for the freedom to enjoy some extras without the emotional reaction.

9. **Eat real food.** Real food is food that your body recognizes and can utilize for all of its nutritional needs. Real food is what your body needs to stay and be healthy, repair, recover, and heal. If the

majority of your diet consists of refined, boxed, canned, and pre-packaged food, do your best to switch to fresh fruits and veggies, lean meats, nuts, seeds, lentils, legumes, whole grains rich in fibre, and dairy low in sugar. Only cut out food groups if you have to. (Obviously, don't eat anything that makes you feel sick or that you're allergic to.) Real food delivers the highest quality nutrients with the lowest amount of waste or unusable materials. For better health, eat it almost all of the time.

10. **Distinguish between physical hunger and mental or emotional hunger.** Eat when you are physically hungry. This will take mindfulness and some practice. Most moms actually overeat in the evening, and most aren't actually hungry at all. Some are, but most aren't. Just like kids, moms like routines and tend to get into the one of putting the kids to bed and then having a snack while they enjoy the rarity of peace and quiet.

Emotional eating because of loneliness, stress, boredom, or exhaustion are also common. So many people reach for food to fill an emotional hunger that it is not capable of filling. Being mindful and distinguishing between real hunger and mental hunger is the key to living a healthier life. This isn't easy, but I promise you that it can be done.

Food is fuel for your physical body. Fill the emotional gaps with a walk, a hot bath, yoga, cuddles with your children or spouse, time with friends or family, time alone practicing gratitude, reading, exercising, or other activities that do not involve eating. Again, this will take time and work but can be mastered.

Last, be mindful of rewarding yourself or your children with food. Food is not a reward; it's fuel for when our bodies need to be fed. It's okay to have a snack, but it's best to do so because you are hungry. Setting up patterns and habits where food is a treat you get for being good can lay a dangerous foundation for you and your children. Let the reward be time together or you getting time alone, but do not let it be the food itself.

Remember, I mentioned this is not about perfection? Well, here's my confession. Earlier, I talked about Zachary only ever wanting his mom and always needing to be held as a baby. Now, at age two, he seems to dislike most people. It's a phase, I hope. We have wonderful childcare providers, but he cries every time I leave him with them to go to work. He's fine after a few minutes but the tears he puts on for me totally break my heart. As I drive to work, I feel guilty as a mom, bad for him and the sitter, and frustrated to have to start my day, every day, this way.

A few weeks ago, I had reached my limit. Remember that last tip I just gave you to not use food as a reward? Well, sometimes us moms need to do what we need to do. Don't judge me, please. I literally pulled out a sucker at nine in the morning, handed it to the sitter and said, "Zachary, there's a sucker for you. Mommy's going to work now." His response? "Bye bye, Momma" Boom, it worked.

I walked out the door with a mom win and a giant smile on my face. He was super happy, and the sitter didn't have to deal with the tears. So, it's not about being perfect all of the time. Sometimes, I break my own rules, and I'm the first to admit it. Since then, I've concocted a healthy popsicle which is working very well, and though I strongly dislike any kind of reward, bribery, or distraction with food, for now, I'm making a concession for the sake of my sanity, and that's okay. Obviously, this is not a permanent thing, and each day has gotten better. He will grow out of it, but until then, I concede. My point? Just do your best most of the time. This really is about progress, not perfection.

Now that you know my ten tips, it's important to note that sometimes you can be doing everything right and still not get the results you are hoping for. When this happens with my clients, I always suggest they check with their doctor and see about getting some bloodwork done. Having the help of a doctor to investigate what more could be going on, such as thyroid problems or lack of nutrients, is very important. Nutrient deficiencies are becoming more and more common and affect most people.

You could either be extremely lacking in one or a few key nutrients, or you could simply be on the low side of normal. If you are low in any one nutrient, your body will not prioritize fat loss. I've seen many clients struggle to lose weight only to discover they are low in iron or B-12 or vitamins C or D or another essential nutrient. This can be frustrating, especially if you are trying hard and following everything exactly right. (And, of course, have given it all more than a week.)

After I had Zachary, my iron was very low, and weight loss took extra-long. My body wasn't allowing the weight to come off, even though I was eating well and exercising regularly. Instead, it was prioritizing oxygen uptake. It makes sense that our bodies will not prioritize weight loss until they have everything they need to function healthily and be safe. Once my iron levels came back up, the baby weight started to come off easily, all 55 pounds.

Side note: You can lose all of the baby weight, no matter how old your babies are. Your body can look and feel even better than it did before you had babies. It will require work and time, but do not believe anyone, including yourself, who tells you that you'll never get your body back. You will and can be in the best shape of your life if you do the work required to get there. It's not too late, and you're not too old or too out of shape. It is possible; remember that.

To get everything your body needs, make sure you follow the nutrition guidelines I suggested. Also, invest in a good quality multi-vitamin for you and your children. This will ensure you get what your bodies need to be healthy and strong and not miss anything that could be crucial for optimal health.

Unfortunately, our food does not have the same nutrient content it once did. Neither does our soil. The bottom line is that we need to supplement. Before you do, do your research. After twenty plus years of carrying supplements, like protein powder, bars, and vitamins in our fitness businesses, I can tell you with absolute certainty, there is a lot of junk out there. Graham and I have sold it and consumed it ourselves. The supplement world is a tricky one to navigate. It is often not regulated, not all natural as it claims, and, in many cases, because it's synthetic, not even recognized as food by your body. I've mentioned eating real food. Eat real vitamins, too.

After years of disappointment, friends of ours, Jessica and Chris Page, who had worked in the fitness business for many years, introduced us to an amazing company. We did some extensive research before deciding because we wanted the very best for our clients and our family and had been let down by other companies.

When I say we researched, I mostly mean Graham researched. He's become quite a research fanatic, which is a giant understatement. Sometimes it drives me crazy, but it's also why I love him. He doesn't settle for anything but the best for his family and our clients.

We're forever grateful to our friends because we finally found health supplements we love and amazing natural household products we can trust. Our son Levi and I are very sensitive to chemical cleaners. Shaklee is the only company we will ever use or recommend again. Maybe you've heard of it. If not, definitely check it out.

After Andrew was sick, we struggled to get his iron levels up. My iron levels had been low for years, and I had tried every kind of iron supplement possible without much success. Often, they gave me awful side effects and made me feel worse. As a result, I wasn't ready to throw him on any of them. When we discovered Shaklee, in just a few months and ever since, all of our iron levels are at an all-time healthy high.

Do your own research, find what works best for you and your family, and just like healthy eating and exercise, which we'll soon discuss, stick with it. Consistency really is the key to long-term success.

With the above guidelines and proper supplementation, you can look and feel your very best and live healthier for the rest of your life. Depending on your nutrition background and diet history, there will be an adjustment phase. Food is not an easy switch, but it has the greatest return on effort.

Instead of overwhelming yourself, pick a few things from this list to implement in your daily living today. Once you've mastered better hydration and consuming a larger variety of foods, for example, add a few more of the guidelines. Take it slowly, but keep moving forward, and in a few months, you'll have made a massive nutrition switch.

The more you can involve your children in these changes, the better things will go. Have them help you, allow them to participate in healthy cooking and baking, and, of course, tasting. Have them start a vegetable garden and learn about growing food. No matter their age, their engagement is the key to this switch working well in your home. The more you involve them, the more they will learn what healthy living actually means. When they see you making healthier choices, they will eventually do the same. Eating veggies will become a part of their foundation. It will be what they do, and as they grow, they will continue to do it.

Nothing brings me more joy than when I see children following in their mother's footsteps. Many of the moms in our group send photos of their children munching on broccoli or brussels sprouts or drinking green smoothies. The impact a mother can have on the health and future of her children is powerful and inspiring. Moms really do have incredible influence to change the lives of everyone in their family for the better.

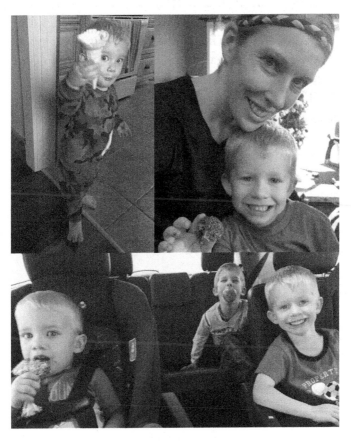

Balance is ice cream and broccoli.

Living in the information era is an excellent time to live. You have access to tens of thousands of healthy recipes at your fingertips. Not only is healthy eating tasty, but it's also trendy, and you will find ideas everywhere. Start looking and never be bored or unsure of what to eat again. Reach out to me any time; I'm always happy to share healthy and delicious recipes.

When you begin to fuel your body well, you will notice you are feeling better, have more energy, and are sick less often. Your kids will be healthier, too. Everyone's health will benefit. You owe it to them and yourself to live a healthier lifestyle and to establish a good relationship with food. You can do this.

That's it, complete nutrition liberation. From this second on, no more toddler leftovers and no more diets and follow some simple guidelines to help you succeed in living a healthier lifestyle. Love your body with healthy fuel, and watch it love you back.

Action Items

No more toddler leftovers. It's time to make time for you, and this means making time to sit down and eat healthy meals. No more running on empty or grabbing random scraps left over from sticky-fingered toddlers (or teens). No more evening binge sessions because you realize you are starving when you finally sit down. This means you fuel your body well because, if anyone's body needs good fuel, it's yours.

No more diets, ever again. Even if it sounds scientific and convincing or promises you'll keep the weight off forever or the before and after pictures are legit and totally mind-blowing amazing, do not do it. Instead, it's time to find the balance between healthy eating and having the birthday cake and ice cream with your kids. It will take time, but if anyone can master adjusting to change, it's you. If you need support, reach out any time. Me and my team of amazing mom coaches are always happy to help a fellow mom.

Follow the ten tips I laid out for you. Take it at your pace. Start with a few if that works best for you and work up to eventually doing most to all of them. These alone will provide you with excellent results.

Develop a healthy relationship with food once and for all. Let go of all emotions surrounding food. Eat when you are physically hungry. Be aware of your nutritional habits and triggers, and remember, no more emotion surrounding food. If you choose to have that bowl of chips, then choose not to have guilt about it or to beat yourself up for it. Carry on with your healthy lifestyle journey, and make your next meal healthy and delicious.

5

Switch #4–
The Fit Switch

xercise. You knew it was coming, and given my passion for it, you can imagine my excitement that we're here. The truth is that you need to exercise, I need to exercise, we all need to exercise. Your body is designed to do it and will love you for it. Maybe not during the exercise, when it's hard, or after, when your muscles are sore, but in the long run, your body will love you for it.

If you want to look and feel your very best, lose weight, increase energy, and be healthy, you need to make exercise a part of your life. Everyone should exercise to maintain a healthy lifestyle, but moms especially should. Here's why: Exercise is proven to be better for stress, fatigue, anxiety, and depression than any medication, wine, or coffee combined. That's amazing!

Stress and moms go together like toddlers and sticky fingers. Fatigue and moms are much the same. Every mom I know experiences both on a daily basis. Chances are good that at some point in motherhood you'll also experience anxiety or depression or know someone who does.

It's important to remember that these things are common, you are not at all alone and should never feel ashamed or feel that you've failed as a mom for being human and having normal feelings. The good news is that there is a lot you can do to help ease the symptoms and cope with the demands of motherhood and life.

There's solid evidence supporting exercise as a means to help substantially lower depression and anxiety while simultaneously increasing your energy and helping you cope with stress. It will also reshape your body and keep it lean, healthy, and strong. I'll say it again, moms need to exercise. If you're not exercising yet, please start now. If you already are, keep going. Exercise is your daily dose of calm. I don't know about you, but with three extremely energetic boys, I could use all of the calm I can get.

The great news is that you do not have to exercise for hours a day or even hours a week to get benefits. You likely don't have time for that anyway, and I understand. You're busy. The other great news is that, when you exercise, your kids are very likely to follow in your footsteps which will set them up for a much healthier future.

Again, I have some simple guidelines to help you fit exercise into your busy life and achieve great results in the shortest amount of time possible. Before that, though, there are two switches you need to make. The first one is the scale switch, which I promise is another liberating switch, arguably the most liberating one of all. The second, which I will get to soon, is what I call the "do it anyway" switch. First, the dreaded scale...

When you first became Mom, and every time after that, your brand new beautiful baby was weighed. The number was probably announced to friends and family and likely celebrated along with his or her name. As you know, what your baby weighs is an important indicator of your baby's health.

As your little one grew, if you were like me, you were hoping to see the number on the scale go up because this meant your baby was gaining weight well, and therefore, was healthy. Chances are good you were excited to tell friends and family that your bouncing bundle was "already fifteen pounds."

My point is that the scale used to be no more or less than what it actually is: one method for measuring health status. In fact, it was once a happy experience. Somewhere along the way, we let it become more than it actually was and gave it more importance than it deserves.

When I was thirteen, I remember being weighed by my family doctor and told that I needed to lose weight. It made me feel awful. This was my first memory of having a bad experience with the scale. As you know, I was already insecure about my looks, so the embarrassment and discomfort about that comment gave me yet another reason to be disappointed with my already disappointing body.

At that time, I didn't have the tools to know how to help myself to become healthier inside or out. I also didn't know how to navigate the awful feeling I had about my current weight. I wish I knew then what I know now about a lot of things, especially about the scale.

The scale holds some pretty incredible significance if you let it. Have you ever been frustrated by it? Silly question, right? I strongly dislike it and not because it shows me a number I don't like, but because we've all given it far too much power.

I've seen happy moms step on it and cry. I've seen people having an awesome morning step on it and allow it to ruin the rest of their day, in some cases even their week, or worse, their month. I've seen people work hard and then allow the scale to end their efforts entirely.

It's a thief. I've seen it steal happiness, confidence, self-esteem, and hard work. I've even seen it steal progress. With one tiny step on the scale, a person can go from being dedicated to completely deflated and wanting to give up. Sadly, sometimes they do.

It has power that it shouldn't have. It has the power to tell you that you're not there yet, not good enough, not working hard enough, not beautiful, not worth the effort, or not worth continuing. It's a liar.

I've told countless clients it's not about that number the scale gives you, and I really do believe this. It's about how you feel, how far you've come, and how much stronger and healthier you are. Making fitness a part of your life is the easy part. The hard part is making the switch from allowing the scale to dictate your mood to using it as one small measurement of overall health.

From now on, I want you to take its power away. You have a choice. I want you to know that the scale is a tool (pun intended). One of many tools, but certainly not the only one, used to measure health, but more specifically, to measure force. It tells us how much gravity is pushing down on us. That's pretty much all it tells.

It doesn't tell us that the reason you are up two pounds is that you've lost five pounds of fat and gained seven pounds of healthy, lean muscle tissue, which, by the way, will make you smaller in size and rev up your metabolic rate. It doesn't tell you that you are retaining water and simply need to drink more water. It doesn't tell you that you've been working hard and can now do full body push-ups and run a few kilometres without stopping. It doesn't tell you that you've gotten stronger, healthier, leaner, faster, or more powerful, and it definitely doesn't tell you anything about your self-worth or beauty, nor should you let it.

Stop letting the scale have more merit than it deserves. Be liberated, and if you use it, use it as a tool alongside measurements, body composition analysis, food journaling, exercise logging, mindset and self-talk journaling, energy rating, and fitness testing, so you can see the entire picture of your progress and not just one tiny little piece.

Stop giving this one tool the power to ruin your day or derail your fitness goals or destroy all of your hard work. Stop letting a number determine your self-worth. Stop letting the scale steal from you and lie to you. Stop letting the scale dictate your success and cause your failure.

If you choose to step on it, please do so knowing the number it gives you is far from the whole picture. It's just one piece of information, and that's it. Once you see that number, walk away with a smile on your face knowing you were beautiful before you stepped on it and are still just as beautiful. You were worth it before stepping on it and are still just as worth it. You were doing great before stepping on it and are still doing great.

Do not let the scale measure your success, self-worth, or effort any longer. Please, start loving yourself beyond a number that in the grand scheme of life means very little. Your children don't care what your weight is. Your loved ones don't care what your weight is. Your spouse, friends, co-workers, neighbors—the people who really matter in your life—don't care what your weight is. What matters to them is your health and your happiness. The scale cannot give you either, and if it can't give you those, it should never be able to take them away. Rant finished. Make the scale switch and never be a victim of it again. This will free you and your children forevermore.

The next fit switch is the "do it anyway" switch. I totally understand and can relate to the struggle of juggling kids, work, a significant other, friends, responsibilities, and life. These days we all have our hands very full. Having kids fills both your hands and your heart and makes for an extra happy life and an extra busy one.

Making time for exercise isn't easy for anyone, myself included. Like many people, I do not have an extra hour in my day that just happens to be free. There is always someone needing me or something to do. On most days, both.

What I do have is a choice, and most days I choose to prioritize exercise. On those days, I feel better mentally and physically. I have more energy, am a better wife, a much more patient mom, and I feel filled and accomplished rather than empty and exhausted. I am not ashamed to admit that I use exercise as a stress coping mechanism and a daily dose of happy hormones. That's what it is for, among other things.

Despite all of this, I still don't always feel like exercising, and you won't either. Many days you will simply have to do it anyway. This means even if you're tired, stressed, cranky (especially then!), unmotivated, sad, angry, or too busy and would rather do anything else—you need to exercise. You will never regret getting a workout in, but you will regret not doing one.

Trust me on this. On the days you feel unmotivated or unhappy, you will come back from your workout feeling better than ever. Doing it anyway makes you mentally stronger, and that strength will help you get and stay healthy.

Doing it anyway will also make you feel proud that you overcame the obstacles, left the excuses behind, and accomplished something healthy for yourself. Feeling proud of yourself is a very good thing and is not something many people can say they often feel. It's worth pushing past your bad mood, excuses, or lack of energy to feel proud.

Some days, your kids will scream as you are leaving and give you horrible guilt. Some days, you will not want to do it at all, and trust me, you will find every valid excuse in the book on those days. Never negotiate. This means the conversation does not even begin. Fight back with that terrorist in your head that's trying to sabotage your workout. Get your fitness clothes on, lace up those shoes, and go get it done no matter what. Of course, listen to your body and be sure to get an adequate amount of rest, but if it's supposed to be a workout day, then it's a workout day no matter what.

The minute I left my first child, Andrew, to carve out some quality me time and get my body back in shape after having him, this unfamiliar, looming feeling of guilt came with me. It was such a strange new feeling, and I had never experienced anything like it before. It was my first taste of mom guilt. I was immediately torn in two directions: one that wanted to stay with my baby (after all, he needs me), and the other that desperately needed some time for myself, alone, to exercise and de-stress.

Choosing to do it anyway has made me a better mom, not a selfish one. I am much better for everyone in my home having had a good sweat session. Sometimes, even now, I still get a hint of that familiar guilt, but I immediately remind myself how much better I will be for everyone that loves me when I return, and I close the door on feeling bad for doing something good for myself. From this point on, you need to do the same.

It sounds wonderful—"just do it" or "do it anyway" or "just get it done"—but the actual doing it part can be very challenging. This is by no means an easy switch for moms—or anyone, for that matter. There are usually a hundred other things pulling you in many directions, and most often, the moment you are ready to get your workout in is the very moment everything comes at you, all at once. The difference between those who really can *do it anyway* and those who just can't seem to get it done is actually quite simple.

MINDSET - Your mindset makes all of the difference in the world when it comes to exercise and getting your workouts in. How you view exercise will determine your mood toward it, and your mood will dictate whether you do it or not. Those who look at their workout like it's a chore, work, or something they have to do, will feel that exercise is punishment. Those who view it as a privilege, their special time, an investment in their health, and something they get to do, will feel as if it's a reward (even though it requires effort and work). Think about this, and then change how you're thinking about it if necessary. This alone will make all of the difference for you.

ACTION - Getting it done obviously requires action, and action is certainly effort, but those who take it have one common focus: the outcome. They actually do not focus on the task at hand (the workout), but they focus on the sum total of workouts (what the workout gets them). They take action because they want the outcome of the action, and they know the action is a necessary means to that end. If you can focus on the outcome (healthier, less stressed, stronger, fitter, more confident, etc.) rather than the task (getting sweaty, muscles burning, out of breath), you too can become an action taker!

EXCUSES - Sometimes the lies we tell ourselves or the stories we believe or the excuses we make get in the way of being able to take action. Countless clients tell me they do not have the time to exercise. They are run down, depressed, in discomfort or even pain, overweight, unhealthy, and at the end of themselves. "No time" is an excuse that will eventually take its own toll on your health and your body leaving you with even less time because now you aren't healthy enough to even enjoy the time you have. Get brutally honest with yourself, ask yourself what excuses you are making, what stories you are telling yourself, and what lies you are believing, and then be ready to set them aside to *get it done*. If I can be real with you, I think moms need to take twenty minutes away from the time they spend on social media and put it into a workout. I promise getting it done will feel much better than scrolling through everyone else's highlight reel.

PRIORITIES - Getting it done *always* comes down to your priorities. If something is a priority to you, you will make the time to get to it. You will find the money for it, and you will move whatever you have to make it happen. Heck, you do this for your children all the time! If it isn't a priority, then it just won't happen; it's that cut and dry. Is exercise a priority for you? If no, then why not? Is your mental and physical health not worth the effort? You may need to re-evaluate what exercise means to you because it is a major investment in your health and your quality of life as well as the happiness and calm in your home.

BENEFITS – You will not always want to do it. In fact, most of the time, it will be a bit challenging to get the ball rolling. You will be tired, you will have lots of other things that seem more important, and you will not always be motivated. This is when you need to focus exclusively on the immediate benefits: how great you will feel when it's done, how much more energy you will have, how much more mental clarity you will have, less stress, more patience, feel-good hormones, etc. Focus on these, and you will actually go through a process of convincing yourself to do it anyway, and when you do, you will feel so much better that you did.

The next time you wonder why you can't seem to get it done, have a look at these tips and be sure you are prioritizing it, being thankful you get to do it, making no excuses, taking action so you can live the healthier life you wish to live, and focusing on the benefits that come from a good sweat session.

Now that you know the switches, I must tell you that making exercise a part of your life does not have to be difficult or time-consuming. Read on for the guidelines our moms live by. These will help you get started and also help you make fitness a permanent part of your life.

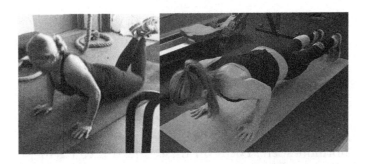

Left: Eight months after having my third baby, Zachary. Push-ups were *so* hard, but I did what I could do, and that's all that matters for you, too. Right: Today, push-ups are still something I struggle with, but my arms are stronger, and the fifty-five pounds from baby is gone, so they are better than they were, and so am I.

1. **Move your body every day.** This is the only time that I'm not talking about actual exercise, I'm talking about daily movement that involves going for a walk, doing yard work, cleaning your home, playing with your kids, or simply parking further away from work and walking to and from your car. Your body was designed to move, and it is healthier, stronger, and more energized when it does what it was designed to do. Incorporate more movement into your life and distinguish between movement and actual exercise. Both are equally important.

2. **Sweat three to five times a week.** It is very important to get your heart rate up and your body warm. It releases endorphins that combat stress, anxiety, and depression, it strengthens your

heart and lungs, clears your mind, and allows you to get stronger over time. Carve out time for three to five sweat sessions a week and make it a non-negotiable part of your day. More is fine, but less is not.

3. **Exercise for twenty to forty minutes at a time.** You do not need to exercise for hours on end to get the benefits. Twenty minutes can count if you make it count. Whatever amount of time you have, work hard, get sweaty, and challenge yourself, and you will benefit. It should not feel easy, it should feel like work. Remember, it's called a workout for a reason. It is work. If you ask me, it's an excellent way to work out all of the mom stress.

4. **Combine strength training with cardiovascular exercise.** Cardiovascular training is important, but it is not the most effective when done on its own. You'll need to also work your muscles to increase your metabolic rate. Spending hours on an elliptical will burn calories, but it will not increase your metabolism, and it will not increase your lean muscle tissue. You want both, so do workouts that involve your entire body and incorporate exercises like push-ups, squats, planks, lunges, burpees, and more.

5. **Stretch.** Incorporate yoga, stretching, breathing, and relaxation into your daily routine. Five minutes of breathing and stretching goes a long way. Tight muscles are weak muscles and need to be loosened and relaxed. Moms need to be

loosened and relaxed! Try to incorporate a few yoga sessions into your week or at least five minutes of relaxation, and trust me, your body—and above that, your mind—will feel the difference.

6. **Work as hard as you can every time.** It is important to get a little out of breath, challenge your muscles, and work hard. You should not look pretty after your workouts, but, of course, you should feel pretty because you got it done. Work as hard as you can and even try to push past your mental limits for at least a little bit of your workout. Obviously, listen to your body and rest as you need to.

7. **Be patient.** This is a marathon, not a sprint. So many people want up-to-the-minute results. They want to click a button and then fit into smaller clothes. It just doesn't work that way. It takes time and patience to see physical results. The great news is that the anti-depressant effect, stress relief, and feel-good hormone release happens almost instantly. You'll walk away feeling better, and in just a few months, the looking fit and being healthier part will follow.

8. **Be consistent.** If you want to lose weight and gain strength, you need to be consistent. Never let a week go by without exercising. Three months from now, you'll be stronger, six months from now, you'll be leaner, and a year from now, your body will be in excellent shape—but it will require you be consistent to keep it that way.

This means you do it anyway, no matter what life throws at you.

Following these tips will help you integrate exercise into your life and will ensure you get the best results in the shortest amount of time. Take note that your children have been exercising since they could crawl and will continue to do so as you show them the way. We were designed to move. Our bodies enjoy doing it, and our minds and bodies will reap the benefits.

That's it, the fit switch made. No more giving the scale power, and from now on, do your workout anyway. Once fitness has become a part of your life, you will be a happier, healthier, calmer, more confident mom. You deserve all of that and so much more, so get moving, mom. You've got this, and we've got you. Reach out any time, and I'm more than happy to help you.

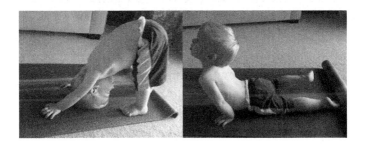

Action Items

Exercise. Move your body regularly because it was meant to move and because everyone needs the amazing benefits that come with doing it. Follow the tips I have laid out in this chapter. Let go of all excuses and pick up this amazing, healthy habit.

Do it anyway. You won't always want to exercise. Many days, you'll have some amazingly valid reasons why you shouldn't do it. Rather than convince yourself not to do it, convince yourself to do it anyway. Make exercise a non-negotiable part of your life. Move your body to keep it healthy and strong. Sometimes, getting dressed for the workout is enough to give yourself that little push. Sometimes, you'll need to be your own motivational speaker.

Make the scale switch. From this point forward, I need you to stop giving the scale more power than it deserves. This may mean you need to remove the scale from your home and stop weighing yourself entirely. In the grand scheme of things, your weight doesn't matter, it's your health that does. Step off the scale and on to the focus of feeling good and loving your body no matter what it weighs.

Mindset. Examine your relationship with exercise. Remind yourself that you *get* to exercise rather than you *have* to exercise. Changing your thoughts and feelings toward exercise will change your actions, too. Remember, this is not a punishment. In fact, I would argue that not exercising is actually the real punishment to your body. Somewhere, there is someone who wishes they could go for a run or lift some weights. Don't take it for granted that you can.

Get moving! Those beautiful eyes look up to you. Choosing exercise as a part of your healthy lifestyle will empower them to do the same. Your workout will become fuel for their future workouts. Inspire them today. One of our codes is "act like your kids are watching." If they were, which they really are, you would finish what you started, you would show up and give it your all, and you would do what you set out to do.

6

Switch # 5– Progress NOT perfection.

The desire for perfection can quickly steal our progress. I think this is why moms are so hard on themselves—they're trying to be perfect. We place huge expectations on our shoulders. We try hard to be the best mom, wife, friend, and everything to everyone. When our hopes do not match with the current reality, we can easily get down on ourselves and even blame ourselves for not being perfect. Us moms have way too much pressure put on us. We've likely all lost our cool a time or two, forgot to pack a lunch or been late for a drop-off or pick-up. The reality is that nothing in life is perfect, including us. The sooner we can come to terms with this, the better off we'll be.

Rather than trying to be the best mom and breaking your back over living up to such high expectations, let's take a much kinder approach. It involves focusing on progress rather than dwelling on perfection. Before you can do this, though, there are a few smaller switches that need to be made. The first one is that you need to stop tire slashing and start fixing flat tires instead.

I can't even tell you how many times I've worked with a client who was doing really well with his or her eating and exercising and then suddenly got side-swiped by life. Sickness, injury, stress, family or financial crises, and all of the unexpectedness of life will eventually happen. Will you let it stop you from meeting your needs and achieving your goals, hopes, and dreams? Because it will stop you if you let it.

Flat tires are bound to happen; they are an inevitable part of life. Unfortunately, they aren't something we can plan for or control, but we can control our reaction to them. Have you ever slashed all of your tires because one was flat? What I mean is something happened that got you off course, and rather than focusing on fixing that one flat tire or moving forward despite it, you slashed the other three tires and sat down in the ditch. If so, know this: you are not the only one this has happened to.

Picture this—say you are eating healthy, exercising regularly, and making yourself a priority. You are on track with your health or weight-loss goal, and then someone you love celebrates a birthday, and you have a lot of cake, perhaps more than the balanced portion. Trust me I get it, cake is delicious.

Rather than carry on with your healthy choices for the next meal, you think, *Well, I've already had too much cake, I may as well have the cookies, too*, and then you also have the chips, the bread, the ice cream, and the wine. Sound familiar?

This is tire slashing, and it doesn't usually end there; it can often be carried into the next day and week. It can land you right back to the dreaded start with the scale weight back up, exercising off track, and healthy eating in the garbage can. Even worse, maybe then you wind up even more down on yourself than ever before because of it all and stop trying to lose weight entirely. This is tire slashing at its finest.

If something doesn't go our kid's way, we definitely don't want them to think that it gives them permission to throw in the towel. Tire slashing is obviously not the way we want our kids to handle life's challenges or obstacles. The reality is that they will mimic what they see, so we need to break this pattern in our own life to also set them free from it.

I totally understand that things can happen that make you want to slash all of your tires and call it a day (or month or even year), but what if I told you tire slashing was ruining your dreams, destroying your progress, distancing you from your goals, and completely sabotaging your life? It's true.

If you're a tire slasher, you need to first realize it, and then you need to stop it immediately. Obviously, stopping is easier said than done, but here's how I want you to tackle your next flat tire: KEEP GOING NO MATTER WHAT! It really is that simple. If you stop, you won't ever get there, but if you keep going, no matter how long it takes, you will get there.

Sure, this may take some serious mind power to navigate through the next obstacle life throws your way. If there is one thing you can bet on, it's that life will throw you some obstacles, but you need to do your best to work around the situation.

Are you injured? Focus more on your nutrition than ever before and keep doing whatever you can to continue moving. Dealing with trauma or crisis? Now, more than ever, you need the mental and emotional release that exercise will offer you. Even if you don't feel like working out, do it anyway. You'll feel so much better afterward. Had too much birthday cake? So what, no more tire slashing. Choose healthy at your next meal and carry on down the road toward your destination. You can do this, you simply have to be willing to do it no matter what.

People slash tires because they are so focused on being perfect that when they make a mistake, they think they need to give up entirely. Instead, try focusing on the progress you've made. For example, say you had the cake at the birthday party and the cookies and wine but your week leading up to that was amazing.

Simply focus on what you've done well, and then move forward knowing that even though you were not perfect, you are making progress and that's what counts. With this focus, you'll be more likely to get back on track and carry on up the road to the next healthy choice. When we can switch our focus to progress, we are more likely to stay on track long-term.

It's time to celebrate progress. What that means is looking back at how far you've come rather than looking ahead at how far you have left to go. When you can change your focus to the improvements you've already made, you'll be less likely to beat yourself up for the improvements you haven't made yet.

To make progress, you need to nix tire slashing. The next switch you need to make is the switch from beating yourself up to lifting yourself up. From here on out, you are not allowed to beat yourself up for anything.

Mistakes are inevitable. You are human, and you are a mom; you will make mistakes. The sooner you can accept that, the better things will go for you. It's time to allow yourself a lot more grace and a lot more forgiveness. It's time to let go of the guilt and constant self-abuse. If you fall, get back up quickly, forgive yourself immediately, and then try again. If you fall, you do not beat yourself up over it.

The first time your child learns to ride a bike without training wheels is quite an experience. I recently let go of the back of Levi's bike seat with feelings of both excitement and nervousness, maybe even a bit of fear. I didn't want him to fall but was worried that he might. In this case, he rode that bike like a pro and was so proud of himself for doing it all on his own.

Had he fallen, though, I wouldn't have been mad at him. It was his first time, he was still learning. How on earth could I expect him to be good at it? And, even as he masters the skill, falls can still happen. News flash, mom, this is your first time at this mom thing. Even if your kids are teenagers, this is your first time as a mom of a teenager. How on earth could anyone, including yourself, expect you to be amazing at it? Even if you're a seasoned mom, falls can and will still happen. Please cut yourself some major slack.

Some days, I really wish each one of my boys came with his own extensive manual and then a daily list of needs. Wouldn't that be amazing? Today, as I write this, it would have been excellent to have a list that told me, "Andrew needs more empathy and gentleness when being corrected. Levi needs more attention and time with you because he's missing you. Zachary needs more playtime and laughter. All three need extra snuggles."

If only our kids came with instructions. We would seriously own the day if it were all laid out just like this. They don't, so sometimes we'll get it wrong, and we need to learn to be okay with that. We are human, and we need grace and patience and forgiveness. We especially need these from ourselves.

Sometimes, like today, that means I corrected Andrew a little too sternly, I didn't give Levi enough attention, and I didn't play and laugh enough with Zach. All three didn't get enough snuggles. Should I beat myself up? No way. Instead, I should celebrate the progress I've made as a mother and keep moving forward and working on the areas that need improvement. Tomorrow will be better. Beating myself up won't get me closer to better. Forgiving myself will.

If you miss a workout, tomorrow is a new day. If you make an unhealthy food choice when you are trying to choose better, simply make a better choice at your next meal. If your self-talk wasn't very kind, make your next thoughts kinder. Do not slash all of the tires; do not beat yourself up. Keep moving forward and be patient, you will get there one celebratory step at a time.

You have patience for your children, and you give them grace, too. I bet you are forgiving when they make mistakes, and I can imagine you would never want them to beat themselves up for something they did that wasn't perfect. Once again, why are you not held to this same standard? You deserve to be. It's time you start.

Your kids did not come with a manual or an easy to-do list, so why do you think you should have all of the answers and have everything figured out? You need to go easier on yourself. Much easier. In every department.

When it comes to the switch—making yourself a priority, loving yourself first, eating healthier, and exercising regularly—it's not going to be perfect every day. But, so long as you keep trying, you will make progress, and that's what counts. What I ask is that you be patient with yourself as you are with your children.

That gap, the one that gets you frustrated because it's so big, the one between where you are now and where you want to be—instead of beating yourself up for it, allow it to motivate and inspire you.

Let it pull you forward, not down. Let it ignite you, not deflate you. Let it fuel you, not flatten you. Respect it. Rest knowing you will close it. (You're a mom, you can do it.) Trust that you have just what you need inside of you to bridge it.

Remember, that gap is just as important as the final destination, arguably more, because the process of closing it will teach you more about how truly amazing, strong, brave, and persistent you are than reaching the destination ever could.

As you make progress, look back and celebrate how far you have come. You may not be there yet (where you want to be as a fit, healthy, role-model mom, wife, friend, etc.), but each day you will get closer, and that is all that matters.

Too many people focus too much on where they are not, on how big that gap is, on how they aren't doing everything right all of the time, and as a result, they get discouraged and stop trying altogether. If you can focus on the progress rather than perfection, not only will you get there, but you'll also experience a lot more joy while you're on the journey. Perfection is the enemy of progress so from this point forward, you're a progress celebrator instead of a perfection seeker.

When it comes to our children, I do believe that even better than the instruction manual I wished for earlier, is our very own hearts. Moms' hearts really do know best when they are attended to. The problem is that moms are not tending to their own hearts anymore, and as a result, they are missing things and then beating themselves up for it.

I suspect if you could take five minutes to relax and breath and sit and make yourself a priority, things would be different in your day. If you could really get in touch with what you need, you would also know what they need as well. We are rushing through our lives and could all benefit from slowing down just a little and being more attentive.

Mindfulness is about slowing down enough to listen. After having that epic mommy meltdown, I realized I wasn't being mindful or slowing down at all. It took a crash for me to learn that I needed to do this. I'm thankful the crash wasn't any worse, and I'm so thankful it happened. It gave my boys their mom back, it was the catalyst that started this movement to help moms everywhere, and it helped me find my way back home. Seeing the lie I had been living has changed my entire approach to parenting and life.

It is no longer "hell hour" in my home at 4:00 p.m. I much prefer "happy hour" now. Don't get me wrong, some days are still very crazy. Some days I'm still very much human, but most days are better because I'm better. My cup is much fuller. I now have so much more to give everyone that needs and loves me.

I do not believe that we were ever meant to shelve our needs and set our own happiness aside in the process of raising our children. I do not believe we were meant to live our lives feeling guilty for taking time to tend to our needs.

Somewhere along the way, things got twisted, and moms got lost. To find themselves again, they need to know that loving their children is a beautiful thing and loving themselves is equally beautiful and important.

I do believe that love is sacrificial. If I could have been the one in the hospital bed receiving blood transfusions instead of Andrew, I would have been in a heartbeat. When he almost died, I desperately wanted to take his place; I love him that much. Every mom I know loves her children that much, too, but I also love him enough to love myself. There are some things we cannot sacrifice if we wish to give our children the best of us, and our needs are one of those things.

My desire is that moms everywhere will realize that their needs, hopes, and dreams matter and are just as important as their children's. I want moms to know that they can still meet their children's needs and have their own needs met as well, it's just that the order has to switch. Most of all, I want moms to know that they can look and feel their very best and enjoy a fulfilled and happy life with kids. They simply must stop believing and living this sacrificial lie. Good moms put themselves first.

Before I leave you to a new life of freedom as a mom, I must tell you one more important thing. Do not, for one second, doubt if you will be able to make the switch. You are determined enough to do this. You may not believe this just yet, but that doesn't make it any less true.

Determination is inside of you. It is not a skill you need to acquire, it's there in you already and has been all along. It was there when you took your first step as a child, fell, and got back up to try again. You didn't stay down and think, *This walking thing is not for me.* You didn't call it quits and never try to walk again. Instead of giving up, you got up, and you kept on trying until you were able to walk.

The average toddler who is learning how to walk falls thirty-four times a day. In our adult world, most people would quit before ever getting close to the thirty-fifth attempt. Most people but not a mom. Moms are different. Moms are the most determined people in the world. Moms don't quit.

You are a mom who got up in the middle of the night to feed, change and care for your little one even though you were completely exhausted and just wanted to roll over and go back to sleep. You've been there through bad dreams and wet beds, bicycle falls and scraped knees. You've waited hours in the Emergency Room in the middle of the night holding a fevered child and then cared for them on no sleep the next day. You've been exhausted but kept on loving. You've been sick but kept on going. That's determination.

You are a mom who is still here, still standing, still trying even when you've had times where everything inside of you wanted to quit. You are a mom who keeps giving even when you are empty and feel you have nothing more to give. You are a mom who would do anything, go anywhere, give everything for your children, and you do. You've been doing it since you held that beautiful child in your arms for the very first time, and I know that you would do it all over again. That's determination!

You, my friend, are the most determined person, so please do not doubt whether you are determined enough to make the switch. Know that you are. I ask that you take all of the determination you pour into being the amazing mom that you are and become that determined for yourself, too, because you deserve it just as much as your precious kids do.

You deserve to enjoy life with kids rather than just survive it. You deserve to be a priority on your own priority list. You deserve to look and feel your very best, to feel like yourself again, to love yourself, and above all, you deserve to be happy.

Take all of your amazing determination and commit to fighting for yourself for a change. I do not promise it will be easy, but I do promise that with each step forward, with each switch, your kids will get the very best version of you, and you will find yourself again. The you that you've been longing to be. The happy you that's been lost in a world of repetitive, tired days and long, lonely nights. The you and the mom you always knew you could be. Making the switch is a process but taking a step toward that process begins right now.

I can't wait for you to realize that you matter just as much as those precious little ones you stay so determined for. I can't wait for you to move forward for yourself with the same grit and perseverance you have for your children. I can't wait for you to start living the life you were meant to live, liberated from self-hatred, dieting, and being the last one to have her needs met.

Believe me when I say that the best is yet to come. How do I know? Because as you know, I've been where so many moms are right now, and thankfully I'm living on the other side. If I can get here, so can you.

Can you promise me that when you get here that you'll reach your hand back to help more moms out of believing and living this destructive, self-sacrificial lie? The more moms we can help the better. Kids everywhere will get their moms back, and moms everywhere will get their happy back, and that, to me, is what the switch movement is all about.

Now, it's your turn, mom. Get your needs, hopes, and dreams down off that shelf on which they've been collecting dust. Step forward bravely and boldly and decide this very second that they are just as important as everyone else's and prepare yourself for the very best life with kids, one that you deserve to have.

This next step is the best one you'll ever take for yourself and your loved ones. Much like having kids, I can't promise you this will be easy, but I can promise you it will be worth it. Now it's your turn to make The Switch, and I'm so thankful to be able to help you do it. Here, grab my hand!

Action Items

No more tire slashing. If you have a bad day, make tomorrow better. If you run into an obstacle, ask yourself, "How can I stay on track despite this?" No matter what happens, do not throw in the towel. You can do this; you simply need to keep moving forward no matter how many nails life pushes into your tires.

No more beating yourself up for being human. It's time to give yourself the same love, grace, compassion, and forgiveness that you give your kids. The next time you feel yourself getting into the cycle of beating yourself up, stop it with a gratitude or "I Am" list, and refocus on why it's important to you to live healthily. I bet one look at your kids is an excellent reminder of why this all matters.

Focus on progress, not perfection. The switch is not about being perfect, it's about being better than you were yesterday. Some days you may need to look back and simply celebrate how far you've come. I've had clients list their progress to show them that even though they may not be there yet, they are closer than they were. You will not be perfect all of the time, and that needs to be okay with you.

Pause. Give yourself five minutes to relax, breathe, and get in touch with your heart and your needs. Doing so will not only bring you awareness of what you need but will also help you clarify what your children need.

Everyone wins when you take some time to get in tune with yourself.

Keep moving forward. The difference between those who get further and those who don't is one simple thing: one group stopped trying, and the other one did not. Keep going no matter what, and you are bound to get there eventually. Remember, it's not a sprint, it's a marathon.

If anyone can do it, it's you. Take the determination you already have and put it toward your needs, hopes, and dreams. Pour that determination into yourself for a change. I promise the entire family will win when you do.

Now, go and make the switch!

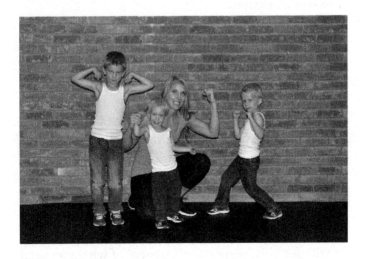

Success Stories
Real Moms
Making The Switch

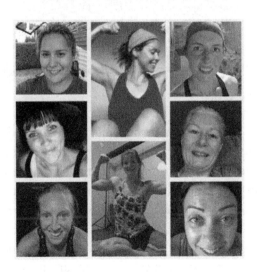

Kirby

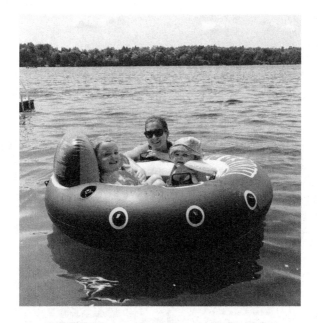

Thank you for introducing this program into my life and the lives of many other busy moms who just did not know if they were ever going to get back to who they used to be; women who had lost themselves amongst the busy hustle of motherhood and were often too scared to ask for help when they needed it most.

Personally, trying to carry a career, create time for friends, maintain a relationship, an intimate relationship at that, with my husband, and complete the endless tasks of mom, I was burning out at a rate that was eventually going to crush me.

Before making the switch, I would wake up with my two children in the morning, brew my coffee, and sit on the couch and watch them play. Key word, watch.

While watching them, I would doze in and out of sleep, dreading the tasks I had to complete that day. I often did not even complete *any* of the tasks on my list and rather would choose sleep. I could sleep all day, and I would still be tired. I was moody, irrational, and just completely unhappy. It was interfering with my life on a whole new level that I hadn't seen coming.

Going from being an active, social woman in my 20s who had a love for friendships, for sport and outdoors, I could see myself, now at 30, getting stuck in an isolated TV and couch world. My mental health was in a state that I never want to revisit again—one of my darkest times where I would find myself often thinking that I can't do this. That maybe, just maybe, I wasn't cut out for this mom thing. Maybe they would be better without me. Those words, those thoughts, looking back now, are absolutely terrifying to me. What was I showing my girls?

Fast forward 22 weeks, after completing the 6-week challenge, and now onto the 52-week program, and I'm down to my pre-pregnancy weight and feeling stronger than ever! I do not sit on the couch anymore in the morning while my girls play. I actually get up before them and have my coffee first alone (mom time!), and when they wake, my attention is solely with them. My energy levels have gone from a 4 to 9.5 out of 10, and my mental health and self-love is the healthiest it's ever been.

Yes, there are days of being a mom that aren't butterflies and rainbows, but I am so never going back to where I was before. I have been lent a helping hand and guided out. And with that, I thank you again. Thank you for putting hours upon hours into this program and for the constant coaching support that delves so much deeper than just the weight loss journey.

I'm a switch mama for life!

Mary Lou

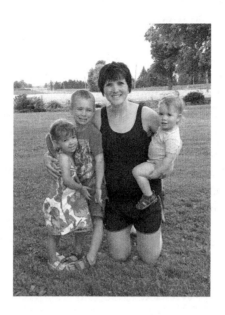

Before I decided to join the Switch Project, I was a busy mom of 3 small children under the age of 3.5. My children are early risers, and my day starts at 5:30 a.m. My days were filled with feeding, caring, running after my kids as well as groceries, housework, making meals, and working as a nurse on top of it all.

To say I was tired would be an understatement. I didn't eat terribly, but it was how I was eating that was a problem. I would drink coffee for breakfast and not really eat a meal until lunch (unless you count scraps left over from my kid's plates). And then I would savor the quiet afternoon naptime by grazing the cupboards and fridge. By the time supper came, I wouldn't even be hungry and would eat very little. Then, once the kids were in bed, I would start my evening binge eating. It became a routine for me. I had trouble getting through my long days because I was feeling so tired.

As the cold weather started to settle upon us, and we were spending more time inside, I started to develop cabin fever. I felt impatient and frustrated most of the time. I wanted to move and be active, and so did my kids. I knew something needed to change. I had been following New U fitness (Alison and Graham's studio) on Facebook for a few months and had seen lots of posts about programs they ran and how successful people had been, but I just couldn't get to the gym to work out. Where would I find the time?

Then I saw the post about Alison and Graham starting The Switch Project. *Could this really be as good as they make it sound?* I thought to myself. What did I have to lose? So, I decided to sign up, and I haven't looked back since.

The tools I have learned around nutrition and eating habits have been life-changing. I started to put more focus on meal prep and organizing my day so that I was eating with my family and not binging on my own. I jumped into the workouts and was surprised at how much I enjoyed them. They were challenging but short and gave me the sweat and high I was looking for. I felt so empowered after finishing a workout.

After only three weeks into the program, I couldn't believe the changes I felt in my body and my mind. I was more patient with myself and my family. I felt stronger and suffered from less fatigue during the day. I even started to notice that my clothes were fitting better. I don't know if it was my attitude, but people started to notice that something was different about me, too. My kids started to benefit from my change as well. They were eating healthier, and they know when I get my running shoes out that it is workout time, and they enjoy doing some of the exercises with me. They are my biggest motivators.

Once the 6 weeks was over, I knew I didn't want my journey to end, so I signed up for the 52-week program. The online support I got from the coaches and other Switch moms has been the driving force that has kept me motivated and inspired all these months. They are there to celebrate your successes and to help you get through the challenges that life can bring.

My physical and mental health have never been better. I still have tough days, but now I put that energy into a workout and share it with the other Switch mamas, and things don't seem so tough anymore. My days are still filled with caring for my family and running a household, but I now have the tools and energy to make it happen. I am so grateful that I took a chance on The Switch Project.

Sheena

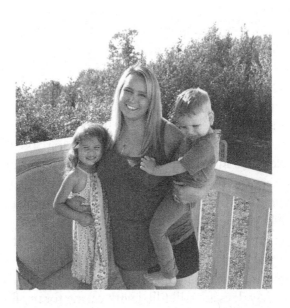

When my youngest turned one, I decided I needed to make a change in my everyday routine. I had postpartum depression after having him. and then suddenly lost a very close family member. I was riddled with anxiety and grief, and I felt an enormous amount of guilt relying on meds to keep me going every day. I decided to try working out to help.

I jumped from program to program trying to find something that fit when a friend posted about a couple I met a few years ago doing a program specifically for busy moms. This seemed like the perfect fit.

I started in December of 2017, and thirty weeks later, I am still loving this program. I have never stuck to a program like I have with The Switch. The workouts are challenging and leave me feeling great, and the community of amazing moms holding each other up is absolutely the key. We push each other and support each other in a way that I couldn't find in any other program.

The support from the coaches themselves is beyond amazing. I feel like they have a vested interest in every single one of us. My anxiety is gone, and I have so much energy. I feel great and have a totally new outlook on my life.

When I was the last on my list every day, I never got to take care of myself until I realized that I needed to stop pouring from an empty cup, and now my family benefits from a happy healthy mama!

Tracey

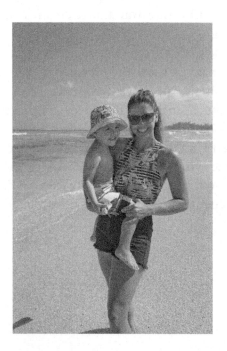

I initially joined The Switch Project as a six-week challenger. My very active son, who at the time was almost three, was not one to sleep through the night. I found myself feeling endlessly burnt out and foggy-minded and couldn't remember the last time I truly felt like myself. It was time to take my life back.

So, I decided to sign up, and I jumped in with both feet! At first, the exercises felt daunting and impossible, but it didn't take long to realize how much support and accountability this group offers via the coaches and fellow Switch mamas. This support was a huge steppingstone for me to continue on with the four workouts per week.

As I write this, I'm on week thirty and going strong, something I never thought possible. Although the workouts aren't easy, I look forward to seeing how far I can push myself and always welcome a challenge with the other Switch moms.

My body has become leaner, with more muscle mass, and I'm feeling stronger with each workout. Along with my physical gains, I've also gained a lot more energy and a positive mindset. I've learnt to make myself a priority so I can provide my family with the healthiest version of myself. I'm learning life is all about balance, and I believe I've found the perfect balance in The Switch!

Karen

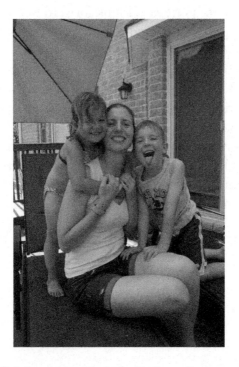

Before I joined the Switch Project, I was comfortable. That's how I would describe it—comfortable. I worked out five days or so a week. I didn't do particularly difficult workouts, but I figured something was better than nothing. I was comfortable in my body and fine with my energy levels. I had come to accept that life was what it was; once you have babies, your body won't completely shrink back, and you will always be in some state of sleepiness.

I joined for one simple reason: I was asked to. I remember the first day on our online group page. I felt like I walked into room full of cheerleaders that all knew a routine that I didn't. They were so excited and ready, and I wasn't. The project held three components: mindset, exercise, and nutrition. Like some people, I don't handle change well, and having to change in these areas was not something I wanted to do. However, I am very stubborn and hate to quit, so I took my time and started to incorporate little changes.

What a difference! Sleepy was no longer a way I described my day-to-day, and I stopped catching those little colds from my kids. With even bigger changes, my body changed dramatically. Without intending to be, I was suddenly back in the body I had in college, and now I appreciate it instead of nitpicking it. I am so thankful for the Switch Project. It was the solution to the problem I didn't even know I had!

Heather

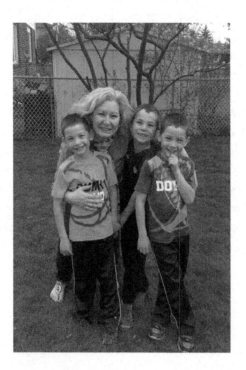

I had all of the excuses: I had three babies in less than two years, I have a thyroid problem, I am a working mom, a hockey mom, a busy mom. I told myself that at the end of the day, after dinner was cleaned up, lunches were made, baths were done, and the kids were finally settled in bed, I just didn't have the energy to work out. Little did I know, or want to admit, the reason I had no energy was because I wasn't taking that time for me, making that time for me.

I had tried many times to get fit. I watched my friends transform their bodies. I wanted it but just couldn't make it stick. The biggest piece that was missing for me was accountability and support. It is hard for me to be successful when my support group lives in a different town. I had no one to get me out on that walk, to be a work out buddy, or to create positive social pressure.

That is what The Switch brought for me. A community of other moms and amazing coaches all in it together. Switch moms encouraging each other, challenging each other, and coaches guiding and teaching.

The Switch changed the way I think about food. Food is no longer for comfort but fuel. Exercise is no longer something I have to do but want to do. Carving out thirty minutes for myself was not hard, it just had to become a priority, I had to become a priority. I am so grateful that I made the switch!

Peggy

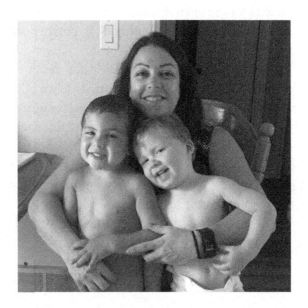

My name is Peggy, and I have two sons; one is 3 years old, and the other is 18 months. I joined the Switch after seeing one of my friends do phenomenally on the program. I loved that everything was online and completely do-able.

In the short time since I have joined, I have lost 12 pounds and 8 inches overall. The energy alone I have gained from this program has been worth it. Mid-day was a struggle, and the first change I noticed was that I no longer needed that caffeine boost or nap. I struggled to complete even one modified push up, and now I can complete several full push-ups on my own!

I always played sports but did not enjoy working out daily; now, it's something that I crave, and this was completely unexpected! My kids have joined in with their own versions of exercise, but the biggest change in them has been watching their food palate expand. My older son hated vegetables and now he *chooses* to eat them.

I love that this is not a diet and that it is simply made for real life. To anyone on the fence wondering if they should join—just do it! It will be the single best decision you make for yourself and for your family. Make yourself a priority again because you are so worth it!

Tina

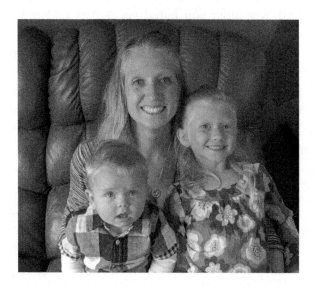

My name is Tina, and I have a 4-year-old daughter and an 8-month-old son. I made The Switch when my son was only 4 months old. In a few short months, I have lost 14.5 pounds and 8.5 inches overall. I've become a happier mom who lost the need for a nap or afternoon coffee because of my increased energy.

Physically, I was unable to complete a single sit-up on day one, but now I can do over 80 of them consistently without stopping and can feel definition in my abs. I have not been this weight or size in approximately 10 years.

The exercises have been tough, but the variety has helped to keep my muscles from getting bored, which has contributed to consistent progress. The biggest change I made was to my nutrition and establishing better eating habits. I continue to enjoy treats but am more aware of what I'm eating and when, remembering that *this is not a diet*.

To all of you starting out, congratulations on making yourself a priority and taking this opportunity to discover how strong your mind and body really are. It's about baby steps and believing 100% that you deserve this, and you are enough!

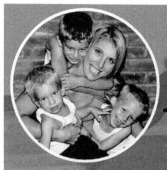

THE SWITCH PROJECT

TRANSFORMATION CHALLENGE

HELPING BUSY MOMS MAKE THE SWITCH!

▌ About us

We help busy moms make the switch from burnt out, overwhelmed and out of shape to confident, positive, healthy role models for themselves and their kids.

Get Energy. Our Moms report going from a 3 to a 9 (on a scale to 10) for energy in just the first 6 weeks!

Workout. No more 2 hour cardio sessions, just quick effective workouts. Exercise smart not more!

Learn The Mindset. You will Learn the 5 Key ideas to make The Switch to healthy living permenantly.

Enjoy Food The Whole Family will Love. We teach you how to eat for life- NO MORE DIETS!

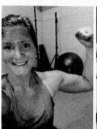
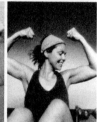

▌ What's involved?

Exclusive coaching from us.

A done for you, detailed training program.

Recipes, meal plan and guidelines to healthy eating.

Mindset Coaching.

Plus, you will be put into a private Facebook group with other moms doing the program and supporting eachother every step of the way!

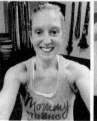
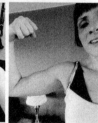

▌ Contact us!

 info@theswitchfitness.com

 @thefitswitch

 @thefitswitchproject

 www.theswitchfitness.com

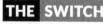

THE SWITCH
P R O J E C T

"A real life, no non-sense, get what you put into it, amazing group of Mom's who get it, and get you! I've gained energy I never knew I had and my family is getting the BEST me. It has taught me perseverance and that when you fall...cause you will...you get right back up one step at a time. I LOVE The Switch!"
- Peggy Procter (Busy Mom)

#IMADETHESWITCH

Acknowledgments

A special thank you to some very special people.

To my parents, Don and Lorraine Wells, for always taking the time to listen to the many things I've written and for always encouraging me to be who I am and do what I do. I am grateful and blessed to have you as mom and dad.

To my sister, Tricia Wells, for being brave enough to step out and let your own light shine. Doing so has always inspired and liberated me to do the same.

To Stacey Ashley for being a true friend who never judged, always inspired me to think on the bright side, and despite living far from me, is always there when it counts. You are an incredible gift to me, and I am so thankful for you.

To my team and family of amazing coaches and one very special administrator, Charlene Cranston, you all help people live better every single day. Your positive impact in our world is tremendous. New U

Personal Training Studio and The Switch Project would not be the same without you all a part of it.

To the inspiring group of moms who have contributed to this book and shared their amazing stories, The Switch Project wouldn't be here had you not jumped on to be a part of this amazing movement and be among the first moms to make the switch. Thank you for reaching your hand back to help and inspire so many others.

To all of the Switch moms in our program who work hard every day to make themselves a priority and support one another every step of the way. Be proud of yourselves; you are showing your kids what healthy living is and their future will be better because you did. Keep up the awesome work!

To Dr. Nicholas Abell, a doctor who trusted a mom's intuition and always takes the time to care; I am forever grateful for you

To Brian Friedman, all great coaches have had a great coach, and Brian has been that great coach for me. Much love and respect for you for helping Graham and I think and dream bigger.

To Jessica and Chris Page, friends, colleagues, and two of the most kind-hearted, generous people we know. Thanks for introducing us to Shaklee and for always being in our corner.

To Judi Stone Photography Studio, a *very* talented photographer who managed to not only keep my boys still long enough to take pictures but also captured the love we have for each other with her lens.

To Candace Eastwood, another very talented photographer and valued member of New U for taking many of the beautiful shots found throughout these pages. I could not have been happier with how they turned out.

To Linh Trinh for giving us the tools to build an incredible mommy movement that's making a giant impact and helping moms everywhere live their best life with kids.

With love and passion, thank you all for your contribution, impact and support.

About the Author

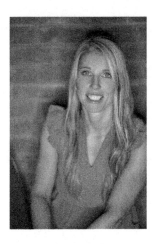

Alison Brown is a mom of three very energetic boys, the founder of The Switch Project, co-owner of New U Personal Training Studio, and a 20-year fitness and nutrition veteran. Equipped with her BA in English literature, her BJ in journalism, and an intense passion for healthy living, she's been writing about fitness and food for years. She is a personal trainer and nutrition coach, the 2008 Fitness Professional of the Year award recipient, an athlete, an educator, and a motivator. Her mission is to help moms everywhere look and feel their best and live their best life with kids.

Made in the USA
Middletown, DE
12 April 2021